Überdacious Living

By
Simone Santivari

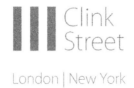

Clink Street

London | New York

Published by Clink Street Publishing 2016

ISBN:
E-Book:

Disclaimer

It is advisable to check with your doctor before embarking on any exercise program.
Yoga should not be considered a replacement for professional medical treatment; a
physician should be consulted in all matters relating to health and particularly in
respect of pregnancy and any symptoms which may require diagnosis or medical
attention. While the advice and information in this book are believed to be accurate
and the step-by-step instructions have been devised to avoid strain, neither the author
nor the publisher can accept any legal responsibility for any injury sustained while
following the exercises.

I would like to thank my parents, Margaret and Simon Thomas for all they have given me and my husband James for making it possible for me to write this book, for his tireless support and confidence in me; for without him this would have been an impossible task. Also many thanks to Jay and Aliyah, our children.

Table of Contents

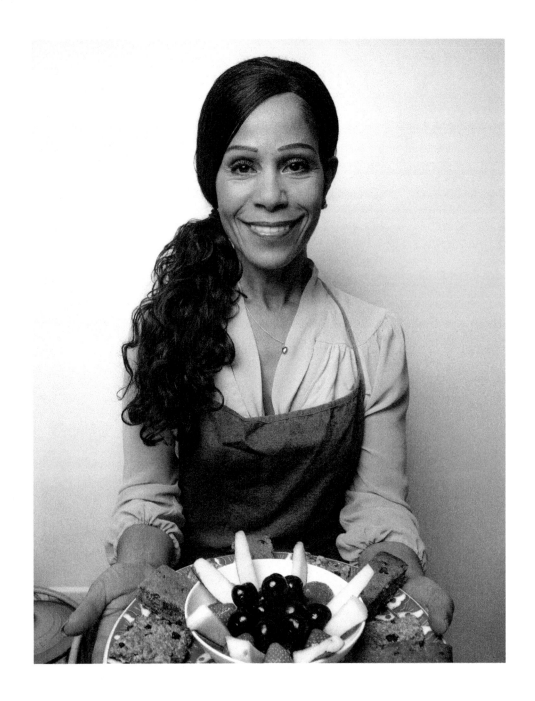

Introduction

It is after a lot of reflection, contemplation, and hesitation that I am finally putting pen to paper. I guess the hardest part when writing a book is getting started. I have so many thoughts and ideas, but most importantly, I want to inspire the reader, not to follow me, but to open the doors to their own mind, explore their own creativity, learn as much from others about life and to see that the universe is here to give us as much as we choose to give it and each other.

I have been fortunate to have met many great teachers and they come in all shapes, sizes, and guises. I hope that I will always be a student of life and be forever curious and willing to learn. We have such an abundance of everything on our wonderful planet Earth, for which I am eternally grateful and endeavour to try to give back each day, where possible. This book is one way in which I can do this, and part of the income from publishing will be donated to charity.

Simone

CHAPTER 1

Spreading My Wings
Doing Teenage Things

I feel greatly blessed and thankful to my parents Margaret and Simon Thomas that from the ages of 11 to 14, I was trained by former British gymnastics champion Margaret Bell, and part of my training as a member of the elite group with my club led to me going to what was formerly known as Czechoslovakia (now known as the Czech Republic) to train in an international camp in Bruno. It was a pretty extreme regimen, but also wonderful, as the camp was in the middle of a pine forest.

Most teenagers are not thrilled to be woken up at 5.30am each morning with strict protocol. Making our camp beds, going to collect yogurt from the local farm, a quick breakfast of rye bread with thinly sliced meat and pickled cabbage, followed by the yogurt – which I did love, because it came in individual glass pots and the strawberry jam was a large blob at the top, even though we had to walk about a mile over green fields and hills to get it! The air was wonderfully clean and pure and the smell of the pine trees glorious. Not a sound of anything other than birds could be heard for miles around. We certainly did not miss the cars or pollution that normally filled our everyday reality and lungs!

Communication with the rest of the gymnasts was limited, but thankfully I was with Carole Gould, another gymnast from my club. As soon as breakfast was over, we knuckled down to training, hard and fast for the whole morning! Lunch was again very simple. Rye bread, thinly sliced meats and sauerkraut. On the odd occasion we would be invited to the trainers' log cabin, where we were treated to the kind of food we were accustomed to eating, and would happily tuck into a bowl of cornflakes with cold milk, which would taste wonderful to us.

In the short time we were there, we were doing moves that we would never accomplish on British soil, and much to the despair of my parents and coach, it was like a wake-up call for me, as I realised we would never get anywhere in the Olympics. Therefore, what was the point in all the training, which took up nearly all my time and life?

The main and most devastating reason I gave up gymnastics was because our Czech host and coach Mr Ruzisckova's son, Steneck, had fallen during training on the vault and had been left paralysed for life. We went to see him at Stoke Mandeville Hospital and it was a truly tragic sight. He had had the skill and stamina to be an Olympian, as well as an amazing physique, but he was now wasting away. He was literally as white as a sheet. The realisation that it could be me lying there really left me feeling chilled to the bone, and incredibly sad for him, and all his family.

Gymnastics had literally taken up nearly all my free time outside of school. I would train every lunch time;

Monday evenings for three hours; Thursday evenings for three hours; Friday, ballet after school; Saturday morning, ballet, then gymnastics for three hours; and Sundays, once a month for the whole day. This left little time for anything else, including schoolwork, as most of the time, I would be going through routines in my head, especially when a competition was coming up.

The thought of telling my parents and coach that I wanted to stop terrified me. I really felt I was letting them all down. My parents for the time and money spent on my training and Dad, also, for driving me to and from the club so frequently. My coach, too, for all the time and energy she had spent on training me. But once I had made up my mind, I dug my heels in, and got on with telling my parents. I remember hiding upstairs when they told my coach.

Once it was all over it left a huge void in my life, but I also felt a sense of relief. Now I could get on with being a teenager and could get on with doing teenage things and having fun and did so with vengeance. My best friend Max, had also been a gymnast at the same club, and we both stopped at the same time and swapped leotards for boys and music and dancing. The trouble was, as with a lot of teenagers, we never got tired of it.

1976 was the year of punk and we were in the right place at the right time to be part of what was known as the Bromley Contingent. We spent our time going round charity shops and jumble sales and finding great ways to make ourselves stand out as much as possible from the norm. With my cropped, dyed blonde hair

and curvaceous figure, I made the most of getting as many heads to turn as possible.

David Bowie had been the main musical influence in my early teens and I still really appreciate him as an artist and songwriter. The look I created was based on the look of his backing vocalist, Ava Cherry, who was incredibly pretty, mixed race, curvaceous and had cropped dyed blonde hair. (I pulled off the look with confidence and the arrogance of youth.)

Bowie gave many a youth the courage to express individuality and not to conform to other people's expectations. Everyone in our group truly worshipped him and I remember the immense and powerful feeling we had going to see him at Wembley, all dressed to the nines: Siouxsie, myself, Simon Barker,

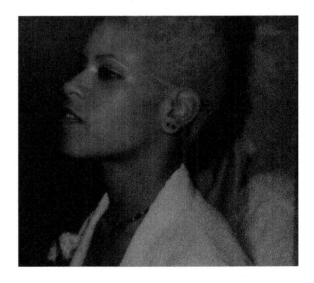

Steve Severin and Berlin (now known as Bertie). Bowie certainly gave it his all and was worth every ounce of our energy, time and money.

During this period, I was fortunate to meet Geoff MacCormack (Warren Peace) who was Bowie's backing vocalist and dancer for many years. We struck up a friendship and he taught me how to salsa dance, for which I am forever thankful. Free lessons from the best!

When we (the Bromley Contingent) met Malcolm McLaren and the Sex Pistols at a gig at Bromley Art College, we were suddenly pivoted onto the London scene. As Siouxsie Sioux from the Banshees and Billy Idol were part of our group, we caught the attention of the press and media in general and were on a few TV programmes, including one with Janet Street-Porter, and also the controversial show 'Today' with Bill Grundy interviewing The Sex Pistols.

For a young 17-year-old it was truly thrilling to have a chauffeur-driven Mercedes with a Thames TV card in the back window come to collect me from my oh-so-conventional and uneventful street. I can't say I was too thrilled once we were in the studio though, and in all honesty was just praying my Dad was not home from work to see me on TV, with The Pistols and Siouxsie Sioux swearing at Bill Grundy; though by this time, the drink we had been given in the studio green room had truly gone to my head, so all you see is me grinning idiotically and trying to stifle my laughter.

I played electric violin briefly with the Banshees. A far cry from the quartet and orchestral pieces I had formerly played. I cannot say that punk music truly moved me, and I am glad I have found my true musical enjoyment, which is much more along the lines of jazz and soulful music.

Around 1977 my father decided to take a contract in Botswana which offered much better prospects, as the long commute he had been doing to get to work was taking its toll and although it was unsettling for the family, it enabled my parents to have a much better and deserved lifestyle. Dad was to be employed as Bursar of the University of Gaborone, Botswana, and Mum would continue teaching. By now, she was also qualified to teach Primary as well as E.S.N. (Educationally Subnormal) children and dyslexic children.

Glynnis, my sister, and I were fortunate to go with them, as the university paid our fares up to the age of 21. Sadly, my oldest sister Arlene did not come with us, which must have been hard on her. Glynnis and I only went for three months, as by now we were way too independent and used to life in London and wanted to feel free and return to our friends and the life we were used to.

Fortunately, I had been lucky in finding a very inexpensive three-bedroom garden flat in Honor Oak. My mother asked if I would let Arlene live there, as she had not found a place prior to us leaving for Africa; so my flat became the new family home as, on returning from Africa, Glynnis also moved in with her friend Barbie as well. I was not particularly thrilled by this, but accepted it was what was to be!

Africa was indeed an eye-opening experience, our first port of call being South Africa. We have many relatives living in Soweto townships on my father's side and things were still pretty horrific and oppressive during this period. Fortunately, because we had British passports, we were allowed access into areas where 'coloureds' and blacks were normally not allowed, such as the better restaurants and hotels. It felt like a really sickening regime. You could cut through the hostility with a knife and the looks on the faces of some of the white South Africans at the sight of us inside what was normally their exclusive enclave shocked them no end.

I distinctly remember, when we stayed at the Hilton in South Africa and I was waiting for the lift, the evil look on this white South African man's face when the doors opened and he saw me standing there. The expression alone spoke volumes to me and I wondered how people could be so hateful. Curiously, even at my young age, I wondered if there was some connection between the South Africans enjoyment for over-salted pig meat to their Boer-like attitude and behaviour. Obviously this is not a generalisation about all South Africans, but sadly that was how I felt at the time. We were glad we were just passing on our way to our parent's new home, which was to be in the university town of Gaborone, Botswana.

Glynnis and I made the most of our Botswana experience and hired bikes so we had some freedom to see the town independently. At least, that was the idea we had in mind. The reality was a little different!

Little did we know just how hot it would be. The first afternoon ride saw us reach the end of the road already feeling like we were being cooked to death by the sun, our faces turning red and blotchy, sweat dripping from us. Even the sun hats we wore were not much help in protecting us from its relentless heat.

Botswana has a very dry, desert-like heat and when you are not used to it, it can be extremely debilitating. Drained of energy, we returned home and ditched the bikes.

Word soon got around that new girls were in town and I remember Mum's excitement when a flash red sports car screeched to a halt outside my parents' new home, with the President's (Sir Seretsi Karma) sons (twins) in it, having decided to take us for a ride. Neither Glynnis nor I were in the least bit attracted to them, but it was a fun experience, though we found them both obnoxious and annoyingly arrogant. On reflection, possibly due to insecurity: they were not good looking but their older brother, Ian, was really handsome, we later found out.

We were fortunate to meet some other young men who were more in tune with us and I started to see Hugh Mogwe, the Minister of Foreign Affairs' son and Glynnis another young man, Ksose, from the prominent Mathews family. Both had been educated in England so were much more on our wavelength. We spent a lot of time listening to great music, going to live concerts at the University, which were outdoors and amazing fun, driving with music playing full blast, and watching the sun set from some very picturesque spots. The setting sun in Africa is a truly wonderful experience, the sky a varying reddy-orange haze and the feeling of being wrapped in the warmth of the balmy air. Glorious!

During the day, we would ask Dad to drop us off at the Holiday Inn, as they had a membership card that allowed us free use of the place, so we spent most of the time by the poolside, showing off, as we loved to dive, and were both pretty good at it.

On one occasion, we were invited out by some older guys, in whom we were not even remotely interested. However, we decided to go along with it. We went home and borrowed some of Mum's clothes and jewellery – my Vivien Westwood bondage gear wasn't what they were expecting – and adding some of her heels to our attire, headed to the door and asked Dad to collect us around midnight.

After dinner, these guys took us to the casino, where, not having a clue what we were doing, we happily gambled their money, and as it got nearer to midnight, gleefully announced that our Father was collecting us, gave each guy a peck on the cheek, and hurriedly made our exit. Not quite what they were expecting. We got outside and burst out laughing. We did not feel bad about it, just thought it was audacious of them to assume we would be theirs for the night. Yes, a little cruel, but on reflection, just the arrogance of youth. Thankfully, with time and increasing years and wisdom, I have grown more sensitive to people's needs and feelings.

Some of my most enjoyable experiences were when I would wake at the crack of dawn and cycle with my younger sister Michelle's puppy dog, Syrup, running at my side, and cycle into the bush. In the early hours, if you sat quietly, it was like watching a David Attenborough TV show come to life. The monkeys would come out to play in full force and it was truly fantastic, watching them swinging from branch to branch. So graceful and agile and also very amusing, naughty and playful!

By the time our three months in Botswana were nearing an end, I was itching to get back to London. I think that Glynnis was as well. There is so much variety here and although we had some fantastic times in Africa, it was just a very long holiday and we needed to get back to living and working again.

CHAPTER
2

Making Music
(and Faking Being It)

On returning to the UK, I knew I would get involved with music again, but needed regular money, as well. Thankfully, luck was on my side. I was very fortunate in having a friend, Max Maltby, who worked for the fashion designer Zandra Rhodes.

They needed extra part-time staff for the Grafton Street shop in Mayfair, and she kindly put in a good word for me and I went in for an interview with Mrs Knight, (Zandra Rhodes' financial / business partner). She was a formidable looking character, weighing a massive amount, and wore huge designer tent dresses and Kurt Geiger court shoes, with her hair always perfectly styled and some elaborate pieces of designer jewellery and of course a designer handbag to match her outfit, completing the look.

She never gave a lot away, in regards to her thoughts, but I got lucky and knew she liked me from the start. So that was that. Überdacious job in hand and designer silk shift dress to go with it. She even loved my cropped blonde hair!

It would have bored me no end to stay in the shop all the time, and I was very happy that they loved the fact I was only too willing to run errands for them. I would be sent to deliver a handbag to Buckingham Palace, or a dress to some rich Arab's pad in Knightsbridge, or sent to Harvey Nichols to collect something for Mrs Knight. It was endless fun for me and I had bundles of energy! I had been on a macrobiotic diet for a few months when I started at Zandra Rhodes, and it gave me masses of energy.

Occasionally when I was in the shop, I was asked to model the dresses for clients (so they could see the visual effect of them on), which I truly loved. Some of the more wealthy clients would buy several dresses at a time, costing thousands upon thousands of pounds.

During this period, I was also singing with The Polo Club, a jazz funk group, and we would often play at The Embassy Club in Mayfair on Sundays. We loved the yuppie, lush atmosphere, and the Buck's Fizz on tap.

We also got to do a number of fantastic gigs and supported Fat Larry's Band at The Venue, Victoria, though the best and by far the most prestigious gig was supporting Ashford and Simpson at the Dominion Theatre, London. Just to hear them in rehearsal was amazing. I felt like a little fledgling sparrow by comparison. They had enormous booming voices, and both, though him in particular, a huge presence on stage, a bit like I am King of the Jungle – you know I am King of the Jungle. Ashford and Simpson wrote many a hit for Diana Ross.

I count my blessings that on many occasions I have been at the right place at the right time. I was pretty forward, when I was younger, and when I went to see the group Blood Donor play locally, I went up to them at the end of the gig and said that if they ever needed a vocalist, to call me. The following weekend, I was invited to record a single with them!

I remember the excitement of driving along country lanes to the studio, Park Gates, in Battle, near to Hastings. Toyah Wilcox was originally booked to sing, but unable to make it, so I was more than ecstatic to be recording the song Dr Who, released by Safari Records.

I remember the thrill of pulling up outside huge electronic gates. I had cropped blonde hair, bright red lipstick, a khaki green boiler suit, tightly belted, and red stiletto heels. Truly thrilling.

Back in London we did a couple of promo gigs at Camden Palace and at the ICA.

We got press coverage in the EMI music paper, and I had a make-up artist, Casey, again thanks to my friend Max, give me a Japanese edge to go with my costume which was based on a kimono design. I was playing electric violin as well as singing, but wish I had felt as confident as I looked. I was actually trembling, and rooted to the spot with nerves. It was pretty amusing that on talking with the record bosses afterwards, they complimented me on my robotic stature at the opening of the gig. Little did they know that I was rigid with fear!

At this stage in my life, I have to admit, I took it all for granted and did not work particularly hard. My main objective at the time was to have fun and be seen in the right place, looking groovy. Now I have learned the value of hard work and I work hard for everything, and it is so much more rewarding.

During the next few years I sang backing vocals for a variety of groups, including Musawa and the Bushmasters – a group from Cameroon – and The Polo Club, and played many London and Bristol gigs, at The Fridge in Brixton, the Embassy Club, supported Ashford and Simpson at the Dominion Theatre, Fat Larry's Band, and was generally out and about on the London scene which was truly buzzing at this time. Steve Strange, Sade, and Boy George were just a few of the faces to become mainstream artists and the flamboyance and creativity was not to be underestimated. Anything went and we enjoyed taking full advantage of the stage of life, at any given opportunity!

I was also asked to appear on a programme called Rock Through The Ages. This was when Channel 4 first started. We were to perform as The Crystals, PJ Proby's group. We pre-recorded Da Doo Ron Ron and another song, and lip-synched on the day it was televised. It was great fun and we were dressed as the original group, wigs and full-length gowns. To our amazement, the audience asked for our autographs after the show. I do not think they cared that we were not the original group so we happily obliged and signed away!

I feel extremely blessed that my first real 'live-in'

partner, Paul Udon, had been a macrobiotic chef. Even as a small child I had an extremely sweet tooth, which did not diminish with increasing years. In fact it got worse once my parents had left London, as I was now free to eat and drink whatever I wanted, and lived on a diet of takeaways and sweets. Greedily I would gorge my way through Chinese from our local takeaway and could easily eat my way through a whole packet of biscuits, guzzle through two or more chocolate bars, washed down with fizzy drinks.

I knew my health was not great, but I still looked OK. It was not until I had been eating healthily for about three months or so, and the natural foods that I was now eating helped me shed unwanted fat and began healing my overindulged pallet, that I felt I no longer wanted the rubbish I had been filling myself with.

When our relationship came to an end, after its shelf life naturally expired (we were together five years), James Plummer, who was a long-term friend I had known since I was 17, asked me out. Really in my heart of hearts, I knew I needed more time before moving on, but went along with it and when he invited me to join him on a trip to New York and Trinidad, I excitedly agreed. I had blank airline tickets (MCOs) that I had not used from my trip to Botswana, so knowing that I could fund it myself was a plus, regardless of the outcome!

New York was a fantastic eye-opening experience and we went to the top of the Empire State Building and visited some funky jazz clubs and went to Central Park. We stayed some of the time at a plush hotel and then some of the time at a grungy dive called the Chelsea Hotel, notorious for housing Sid Vicious and The Stranglers, just for diversity!

A friend of James's was living in New York at the time, the Honourable Oliver Foot, nephew of the politician, Sir Michael Foot, so we spent some of our time with him. James's ex, Susie Smythe, was also there at the same time, so we made an odd foursome indeed. Sadly, Oliver has since passed away.

CHAPTER
3

Me - Myself - Health

I know that in my early 20s, I was borderline anorexic and bulimic. Not all of the time, but in spurts and starts. It was like three steps forwards, two steps back. The information I was feeding my brain, and wanted to sustain, was almost like an impossible task for me to assimilate all at once and trying to let go of all my old habits had to be done at a more gradual pace. I want to apologise to family and friends for the pain and stress I put them through. If only I could have spoken to my younger self and given her guidance! I also wish to thank Glynnis, for trying in vain to help me. Some things we do have to just learn for ourselves and it can take time. I guess that not having parents here in the UK did not help. There is no blame though as I had chosen to return to London and really have no regrets. Going through all I experienced also gives me an inner understanding of others who are suffering; if life were only a bed of roses, we would not be able to understand others' pain and sorrow, so I do give thanks for all that I have experienced!

Turning everything around is very empowering. I think from a young age, we are led to believe that the doctor is there to cure all our sickness, aches and pains. I have learnt that it is better to help ourselves where possible and with the internet, there is so much information available to us that, unless we are seriously ill, the self-help approach is usually advisable. Often the chemical medicines prescribed have serious side effects. I choose to google homeopathic remedies and dietary supplements, which have no side effects, and in my experience, work!

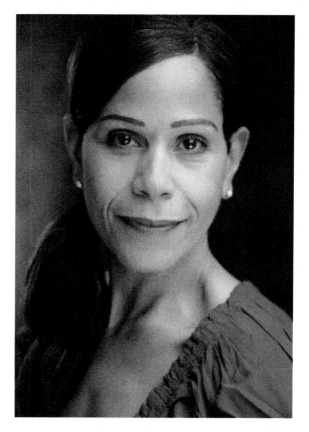

CHAPTER
4

Coming Out Of The Woods (Motherhood)

I did not have my son Jay until later on in life; another blessing! I was really not good mum material until my early 30s, though totally ready by the time he came into this world when I was 33 years old. I had a new healthy regimen, and thankfully was able to maintain this lifestyle while bringing him up. I know for sure this was one of the reasons why he was never ill. The only time he was ever sick was once as a toddler, when he caught a virus, and then again when he was around five and was invited to one of his school friends' parties. He was given lots of sweets and rich cake, which, on returning home, he instantly threw up and was fine again! Not that he did not have any sweets, but generally I made my own biscuits and cakes using less and more natural sugars, i.e. agave nectar or fruit sugar and bought him sweets from the health food shop.

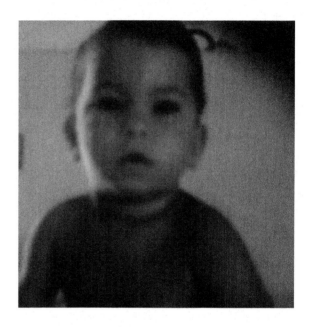

On returning to the UK from Spain with Jay, who was three years old at the time, I was very fortunate to get work in Greenlands, a health food shop in Greenwich Market, which is owned by Steve Chong, a very likeable Chinese man. I call his shop Aladdin's Cave, as it is always so well stocked; in fact chock-a-block, full to the brim with every conceivable health food product imaginable. It is fantastic how he manages to fit everything in it.

It was a great place to work, as it meant I could take Jay to school and be home in time to collect him at 3.30 pm from school, get a discount on all the wonderful products and also, having a genuine interest, be very helpful to the customers.

Jay and I usually went to the park on our bikes after school. A little TV is OK but I was much happier with him getting fresh air and exercise. He was also given a baby Mac computer by our friends Sue and Pete McNeill, and would enjoy writing stories on it from the age of five.

Jay was an extremely bright and attractive child and went to contemporary dance classes from the age of three at Greenwich Dance Agency and played guitar from age five. He was also very happy, good natured and popular and enjoyed cycling, rollover blading and loved playing his guitar. He has grown into a very competent, attractive young man and continued to pursue his love of music; he is now working as both producer and sound engineer and I am very proud of him.

Making the separation from Jay's natural dad, Peter Heigl, was difficult, but on reflection, it was for the best. People change and from a mother's perspective, I knew that Jay would have a better life in London. It was a sad time and hard to make the break, but it was the wisest thing I could have done under the circumstances.

On returning to London, James, of whom I spoke earlier (whom I had had a brief relationship with in my early twenties), and I got back together. He has a daughter, Aliyah, who is a year older than Jay, so we formed a ready-made family.

Aliyah, my stepdaughter, has grown into a mature, intelligent young woman. She is now 26 and we have a lot in common. She also has a preference for a vegetarian diet. She is very attractive and has a successful career in private equity. She enjoys spending a lot of time travelling and like most young women, enjoys fashion and has recently got into fitness and has a fantastic figure. James and I are both very proud of

Aliyah and Jay. Not just because they are bright and successful, but also because generally speaking, they both have kind, empathetic and helpful natures.

I was fortunate in securing a council flat for Jay and myself when we first returned to London; though it took around six months to get it, this is a relatively short time. I felt it necessary for us to have our own place so as to give us space and James freedom to decide for himself and in his own time where our relationship was going to go.

Fortunately, Jay's nursery school was literally five minutes away and the primary school he was to go to was next door to the nursery. He was very happy at both, which was a huge relief to me. My parents were in Africa so I did not have much assistance in bringing up Jay. That is, until his father Peter decided he wanted to live in London. On moving here, he became a great help when I was working, as he would often look after

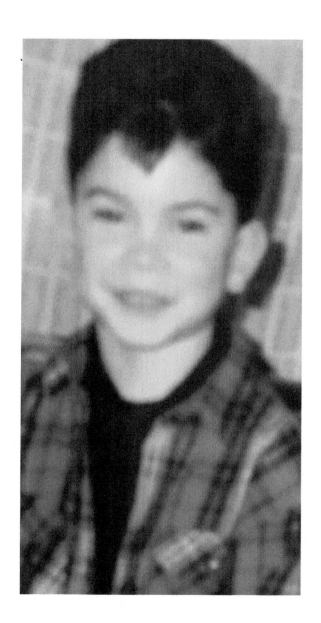

CHAPTER
5

Competition Queen, Reigns Supreme!

One thing we did not have was a lot of money, so I decided to enter competitions to see if I could win us a holiday. The very first one I entered was in Chat magazine. The question was; 'Where is Lake Garda?' I immediately put a card in the post with the answer and was delighted when I was told I had won a holiday for two. Jay and I had a wonderful time and the trip also included a coach trip to the Dolomites and Venice! Truly amazing, though the winding mountainous roads were pretty hair raising and I remember one of the female passengers almost in tears. Jay took it all in his stride though and was adored throughout the holiday, by the other passengers and tourist guides alike.

Shortly after returning to London, Jay and I were in the kitchen one morning and they announced on the radio (Magic FM) a competition to win a holiday to the Philippines. The question was, 'where is Miss Saigon being shown?' I immediately ran to the phone and left my message on their answer machine. It was the Theatre Royal, Drury Lane. I completely forgot about this competition, and a week later when I listened to my messages, I got a huge shock when I was told I had won a holiday for two to Dakak Beach resort, in the Philippines, plus ten tickets to see Miss Saigon at The Theatre Royal. I literally leaped around the room with joy, whooping with delight!

As well as working in the health food shop, I was also doing an Access to Music course, which gave me little free time outside taking care of Jay, so this holiday was an amazing gift, for which I will be forever thankful.

Jay and I had a fantastic time and the Philippine people are so warm and friendly, they made it really special. At first they thought we were wealthy guests but when they realised that I had won the holiday, they took us under their wing and invited us to their village on horseback, got us fresh fruits and welcomed us into their homes. Totally awesome! They have very little money, but a huge amount of love and compassion. One of the best experiences of the holiday was riding along the beach in the shallow water on horseback. Totally magical.

When you win competitions, it is a kind of supernatural empowerment and winning two holidays was incredible but when I won our third, in the space of one year, it felt totally like divine intervention. My mother says it was my reward for working so hard to give Jay the best life that I could give him.

The third competition was via OK! Magazine. I had just dropped Jay and Aliyah off at the dance agency and I went over the road to what was then known as Somerfield Supermarket. I did not even buy the magazine, but on the cover, it announced a competition in conjunction with Heart 106.2, Monday, Kid Jenson's Drivetime. I flicked through the magazine excitedly, trying to guess what the competition would be about, then realised the cover gave me the biggest clue. Posh Spice and David Beckham donned the cover in all their wedding finery. It had to be on them, but trying to guess the question they would ask, that would win me the holiday, seemed futile. I just planned to make sure that I was tuned in on time on Monday afternoon. Lo and behold, heart beating nine to the dozen, there I was tuned in and as soon as they asked the question, I got through! I gave my answer! Then there was a pregnant pause in which it felt like my heart would literally leap out of my body! 'Simone Thomas of Greenwich has the answer! Posh Spice and David Beckham's going away outfits were lilac! Simone has won four tickets to Florida, Disneyland, plus car hire, hotel and flights!' Wow, wow, wow. I was incredulous. It felt totally surreal. It was wonderful to be able to tell James and invite him and Aliyah, as usually it was James paying for all of us.

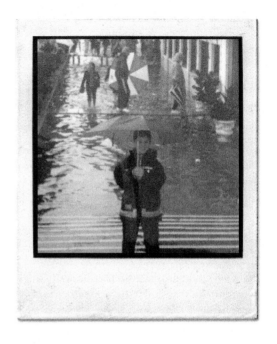

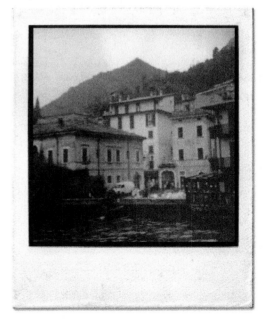

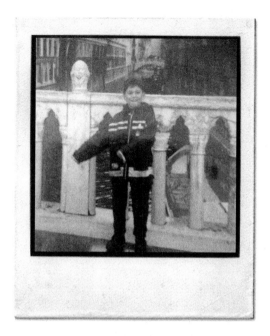

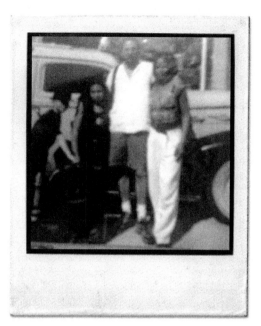

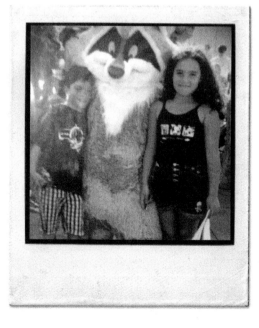

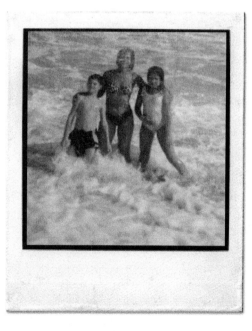

CHAPTER
6

Action! Shoot! Smile For The Camera!

Many people had suggested that Jay should model but I was pretty apprehensive about it. What if he became an arrogant brat? At the same time, I felt that it would be unfair to not give him a chance. He may love it and not be affected in negative way. One of the other boys in his class at primary school was doing some modelling and I got talking with his dad, who gave me the agency details.

Norrie Carr is a well-known children's agency in London. I sent them a photo of Jay and we were invited in for an interview. They then did some test shots and shortly after, he was on the books. The good thing with children is that they live pretty much in the moment. Jay would go for a casting and not think about it again. If he got a job, he would do it, then forget about it. Perfect! I had been worrying for nothing. It was a great way for Jay to learn the value of money as he could see for himself tangible rewards, like buying himself an effects pedal for his guitar and a computer. He continued to model until he decided he no longer wanted to around the age of 16.

It was through Jay's modelling that I started working in film. Initially just as a supporting artist, but as I have a lot of skills, I have secured many walk-on and featured roles. Over the years, I have had a great deal of fun and made many good friends. The roles have varied greatly, from rollerblading in the film Wimbledon to recently playing a debutante parent in Beauty in the Beast. My husband James, says it is the perfect job for me, as I do really love clothes and dressing up; well, mainly when the costume is one that I really like. The worst part of the job is if you are in period costume and they put you in a manky pair of shoes. I take leather liners with me now I know better, and slip them inside.

One of my favourite films was Love, Actually. We filmed scenes in beautiful London locations, dressed beautifully and the weather was fantastic. Between takes we lay on the lawn playing Scrabble and during the wedding scenes, listened to the wonderful quartet that played and the choir and the soloist, who was fantastic. Total bliss!

I also enjoyed Thunderbirds for completely different reasons. Our characters were meant to act like we were drowning in a pod, over the Thames. In reality we were shooting the scene for a week at Pinewood Studios. It was action-packed and under our ordinary clothes we wore wet suits. The pod had a ledge in it where you would normally sit, but as it was meant to look like we were drowning, as soon as the crew started to fill it with water, we had to jump onto the ledge and make out we were struggling to survive. Great fun, as there was about ten of us falling about and on top of each other. We were all pretty exhausted by the end of the week though and glad it had come to an end.

Straight after that finished, I was off to Minorca with my family, the Dohertys and film crew, to film the very first in the series of Holiday Showdown. This turned out to be way more controversial than we had ever imagined it would be. When we were initially asked to do the show, the production called it Holiday Hotspots, which is very different to Showdown. We also liked the idea that we could choose our holiday location and that they would pay for everything, and we chose Jamaica, where James has a house and many friends.

You do not meet the other family, or even know where you are going, until the plane lands. The other family were not people we would normally hang out with and absolutely would not go on holiday with them, as our differences were so great. You could say as different as chalk and cheese.

On the first meeting, Mr Doherty was smoking in a room with our children in it, aged 10 and 11 years old. I find this abhorrent and ignorant, and I think most caring parents would feel the same way. He also said that Aliyah, our 11-year-old, could have two glasses of wine a day like his daughter. Makes you wonder what was the matter with the man. How dare he say what our children could or couldn't do? But in hindsight, maybe he was just nervous because of the cameras.

I do hold the crew responsible for a lot of the bad vibes, though, as we had to make a video diary each night and after they saw our first one, where we tried to give a neutral opinion about the family, they really tried to stir up trouble and said that if we didn't say what we really thought about the Dohertys then we

would look really stupid.

Our time spent with them, in all honesty, went from bad to worse. They gorged on junk foods all day, whereas I have a preference for healthy eating and like to feed my family good quality, healthy food. As the first holiday was their choice of location, they controlled the budget. I went to the shops with them to try and get some healthy food and water in the trolley. When I asked Kim (Mrs Doherty) if I could get a large container of water, she put her hand on her hips and said, "What do you want water for? If you want water you can get it from our apartment!"

I was totally astounded and retorted, "What if I want water in the early hours when you are sleeping?" Fortunately that silenced her and I left the supermarket having purchased with money from her budget a loaf of brown bread, cucumber, tomatoes, tuna fish, avocado, some fruit and water. Enough so we would not starve. Their trolley was groaning with Coca-Cola, bacon, eggs, white bread and a whole load of other unhealthy foods. Their choice entirely, but they just could not understand why we did not want to go and have a fry up at theirs each morning for breakfast, followed by chip butties for lunch and why we were not thrilled by the horrible looking buffet provided by the hotel, comprising limp-looking lettuce, tinned sweetcorn, mass-produced coleslaw, white bread, more chips and a whole load of processed, barbecued meat. Even their idea of a treat outside the complex was fish and chips! We did eat out once in a fairly nice restaurant, but their budget would not stretch to eating out again, which was hard on them and partly

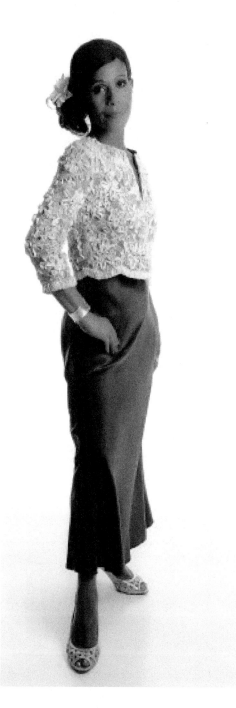
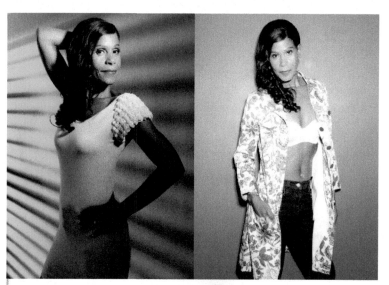
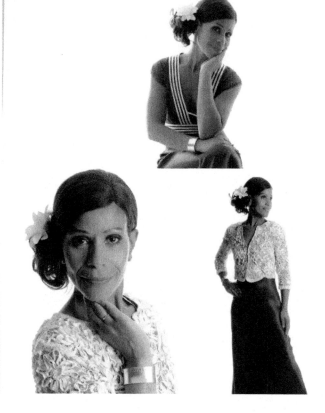

designed to humiliate.

When we arrived at our location in Jamaica, it felt like we had arrived in heaven. We had our own chef and butler and they had got in all the foods we enjoy and when we went out for the day, the dear man would prepare a hamper of food for us to take with us. Everything he prepared was amazing but the Dohertys had to spoil it by moaning and groaning that it wasn't food that they were used to eating. The chef had been trained in America and could cook anything. They say ignorance is bliss, but it just seemed really sad to me that they could not see they were plain rude and small minded.

Of course a lot of the circumstances of this holiday were out of our control. The TV production company set it all up in order to make extreme viewing and secure viewing rates. The Dohertys came out the worst, for this manipulation meant they were given a very small budget for their holiday, whereas we had a huge one. If they felt angry and upset, it is understandable. The problem is that they could not see it for what it was and whenever we warned them that they were being set up, they were completely in denial and went on about how the crew were their friends and had been to their house.

I am quite sure they were of a different opinion once they saw how the show that had been cut and edited and really exploitative, showing them swigging drink after drink from those long necked vases you get in Spain, the husband swearing as he looks out at the beautiful horizon and saying, "Beautiful sea until I piss in it!" Truly gross. We were very happy when filming ended. We decided to give back our return flights

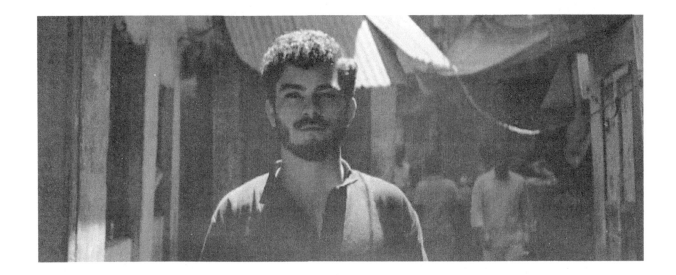

to the production company and stayed on to have a lovely holiday without them, the Dohertys or cameras.

James had built a house in Jamaica several years prior to filming; it had, admittedly, got extremely run down, but that was because James had let one of the local lads who had help build it stay in it, and he had filled it with no end of rubbish and the sanitation left a lot to be desired, so we stayed in one of the guest houses along the water front, with a lovely jetty. I love the water so this filled me with joy as I could go for long swims whenever I chose to. We also went river rafting, boating and horseback riding. James has a friend, John Baker who has a recording studio close to where we were staying, called GeeJam. A lot of major recording artists use it including No Doubt's Gwen Stefani. We enjoyed being shown around the place, which was truly beautiful. A great place to record!

It took a few days to remove all the negative thoughts that filled our heads from our film experience but we soon got over it and had a fantastic time.

I have been with most of my agents for over 16 years: Screenlite, Ray Knight, Casting Collective, the modelling agencies Norrie Carr and Looks London. Most recently I have got an acting agent, Longrun Artistes Agency, and finally Piece of Cake. I am also with Spotlight, Equity and Bectu. If you want to work professionally in this industry it is worthwhile joining reputable agencies that are reliable, just as it is important for the artist to be professional and punctual, as reputations are at stake. The hours can be very long and gruelling so I always take music and something to read between takes. Having a large wardrobe of clothes helps, so whatever character you are playing, you always look the part.

Going to castings can be a bit daunting at first, but the more you go to, the more natural they seem. I know a lot of people do not like them, but I really enjoy them as I like a challenge and the rewards are great when you are chosen for a featured role. Nothing ventured, nothing gained!

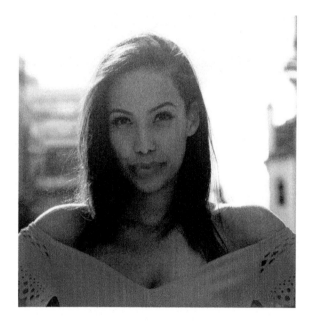

CHAPTER

7

L o v e   a n d   M a r r i a g e

James proposed to me several years after our return to London and I have to say that it came to me as a very big surprise. We were out and about in London at the time and went to the ICA, which is an art institute at the entrance to The Mall, Green Park, where Buckingham Palace is, and he went down on one knee, and asked for my hand in marriage. Of course I agreed. It had been a long time coming; roughly seven years. I was delighted that the courtship had moved on and we spent the next year making plans for our big day.

We then rented out my flat and Jay and I moved into Maze Hill permanently; though we had spent half our time there previously, now it really felt like home.

The wedding came and went in a flurry of excitement and a huge amount of preparation. Thank God, James was totally on the case. I want to also thank Sandy Willimot for all her help and also Richenda (one of Jay's school friends' mums). She lent us an Aston Martin for the wedding, and also a huge thanks to Rene for the Rolls Royce. His wedding present to us for our big day! Also a massive thank you to my parents for my beautiful wedding dress. We got married in St Alfege Church in the centre of Greenwich, which made it very poignant and special; all the history connecting it to our house, as Hawksmoor designed the church, and also the mausoleum in our garden. James looked fantastic in his silk wedding suit designed by his friend,

the designer, John Pearse.

One of James's closest friends, Geoff Holland, was our best man, and did a sterling job along with other friends who helped made the day very special: Spencer Muirhead, Burro and Abedaye, some of our Jamaican friends.

We decided to have our reception at home and I made most of the food with the help of our friends, and also a huge thank you to Steve Chong, as he gave us lots of food from his health food shop, Greenlands (where I worked part time) which I then prepared at home; and thank you to the wonderful baker who made our wedding cake which was organic, low in sugar, but totally delicious. She had glazed dried fruit on top, which made it look like shining jewels and it was three tiers high. Wonderful and very delicious!

Jeanie Missen and my mother, Margaret Rose Thomas, also gave wonderful readings, and great thanks to the choir and musicians who helped make our day very special.

Both mine and James's father, Roy Plummer, as well as Geoff Holland, gave brilliant speeches, which moved some of the guests to tears. A very huge thanks are due to my mother and Michelle and everyone else who helped and also cleaned our house after the reception, when James and I left to go on our honeymoon. It was an occasion that came together like magic and with Anna Malni who took some fantastic photos, our photographer at the helm (who worked hard all day), and also thanks to Javier Molina, we have some great photos, capturing the day. Also our wonderful neighbours, at the time Sue and Pete, who kindly made a video for us. Really amazing! James has a friend Alan Williamson who lives in Uganda and he sent 200 red roses, which we adorned the place with. Really beautiful!

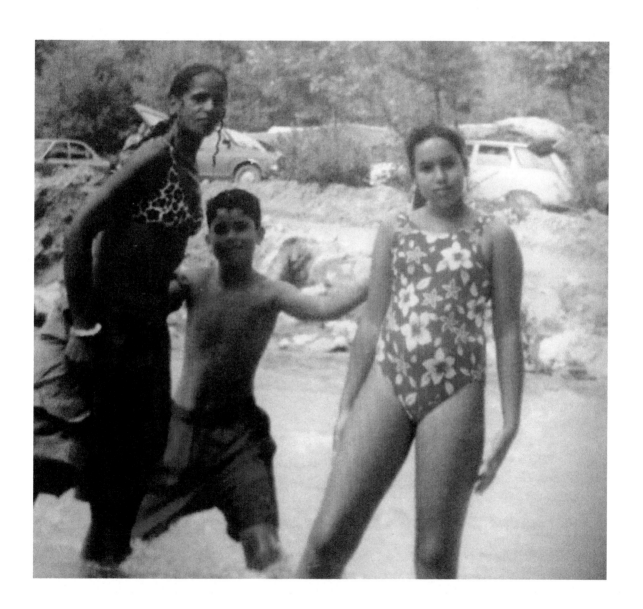

CHAPTER
8

40 Maze Hill

It was indeed a house to be remembered; an incredible property with unique and individual character that James had purchased at the height of his success, around 30 years ago! In fact, it was his girlfriend at the time, Clare, who found the place. James was in a great place financially and asked Clare to look out for property to buy. Luckily she has great taste and Maze Hill was a superb find. Although in pretty bad condition at the time of purchase, it was a former surgeon's house overlooking Greenwich Park, with fantastic views and amazing history. Surrounded by a high walled garden with a private entrance leading into the park, a mulberry tree in the centre of the garden gave it unique character (this tree, along with two others, was brought over for King James; the other two are at Charlton House).

We also had a mausoleum at the end of the garden, which we renovated and turned into a music rehearsal studio. A large outer building at the end of the garden was turned into a health studio/gym. As a grade II listed building, we kept all the original features of the property and at the back of the house, on the first floor, were French doors and an ornate balcony overlooking the back garden. On the ground floor, elaborate Victorian balustrades surrounded the patio. It had previously been owned by former Prime Minister, James Callaghan. It truly was James's castle and dream home and it was where Cheryl, the mother of his daughter, gave birth to Aliyah, so poignant memories that cannot be replaced remain in the very walls and foundations.

It was very sad for James to have to let go of the place but at the same time a godsend as he was now in a financial position not to have to worry for the rest of his life. With good investments in place, thanks to his friend Charles Style (who is a property developer) we were able to buy our new home outright, and pay off any outstanding debts. A great feeling!

Lucky Jay (Has A Winning Way)

Jay's primary school was having a competition in conjunction with Blue Peter. The children were asked to write a paragraph on what the Millennium meant to them. The winning entrants would be invited to open the Dome for the Millennium celebrations.

Thirteen children were chosen and Jay was one of them. They had several rehearsals, which they found to be enormous fun and were given Nike clothes and trainers for the opening ceremony. Many important delegates were there, including the Queen and the Prime Minister, and after the opening all the children were invited to shake hands with them. Jay truly loved the whole experience and I felt a great deal of motherly pride seeing my son run down the centre aisle of the dome and pulling the cords that opened the curtains as the opening music struck up and everyone stood to attention. It was a flawless performance given by all the children and I know that his headmaster, David Suttle, must have felt just as proud as us parents. I think that God works in wonderful and mysterious ways because at Jay's secondary school he was again given an opportunity to shine above the norm. Jay was fortunate to get into Haberdashers' Aske's, which was, at the time, one of the best non-fee paying schools in London. I decided to get him extra tuition before taking his entrance exams and I think this was a great help as they gave him test papers in his extra tuition classes, which I think gave him a lot more confidence. We were totally thrilled when he was told he had a place. After he had sat his entrance exam he exclaimed: "It's just like Happy Potter; I want to go to this school!" The interior design was very old fashion and did resemble Hogwarts.

He started singing in the school choir and also continued with classical guitar and also rock guitar lessons. Luck would have it that one of the mums worked at a recording studio that The Darkness (a pop group) were recording at, and suggested that they approach Haberdashers', as they wanted some kids to sing on their Christmas single. The choirmaster was a perfectionist and got the best out of their voices, always making sure they gave flawless performances. Jay was one of them. He thoroughly enjoyed the whole experience: rehearsing, interviews, performing live concerts and on Top of the Pops and to top it all, royalties, which he still gets to this day!

I think it did go to his head for a while, but fortunately he settled back down again and after floundering around a bit, on leaving school, went to SSR, a private college in Camden, where he got a half scholarship and began his training as a sound engineer/music producer. He is now enjoying some fantastic gigs in and around London and also produces artists at his home, where he has his own studio.

CHAPTER

9

Living With Disability (Finding Inner Sensitivity)

Sadly, my husband James was diagnosed with Multiple Sclerosis several years ago. He is naturally an alpha male type personality, who ran his own company and was very successful. He used to run around the whole of Greenwich Park every day. Before he was diagnosed, he would come back from his run from time to time saying that he had fallen over. This seemed pretty odd to me and I suggested he go to the doctor, but he was not keen to, and being an unwilling patient at the best of times, ignored it; that is, until we went for a long walk in the woods with my son Jay, and his legs gave way beneath him!

This time he listened to me. On returning from the doctor, he said he had sprained his ankle. Eventually, he persuaded them to give him an X-ray. Three months later we got the results. He had fractured his ankle. He also got the results from an earlier MRI scan. He was diagnosed with MS.

This did not surprise me, but the realisation for everyone was pretty devastating. We are all still trying to come to terms with MS, the effects on his body and mind (of course) being terribly stressful for James.

There is still a lot that needs to be understood about this condition. Is it hereditary? It is an autoimmune disease, which means the immune system is attacking itself? They do not know whether people have a genetic weakness which means they are pre-disposed to get this condition, though they do know that it is stress related and that the myelin sheaf which is located in the spinal column, has worn away in those with Multiple Sclerosis and that they have lesions on the brain.

At this present moment, to date, there is no cure. God willing science will advance in the very near future. Possibly stem cell therapy will be the answer.

Life goes on though and the best way we have found of dealing with it is by taking one day at a time and trying to concentrate on the positive and not dwelling on the negative. If one looks too far ahead, the imagination can run riot and imagine all sorts of terrible and horrendous situations, whereas by taking one day at a time and living in the moment we can cope with most things, even though it can sometimes be very hard to deal with.

Most people, unless living with a person with a severe disability or handicap, have no idea what they have to deal with on a daily basis. Everything that able-bodied people take for granted is basically bloody hard work. Just getting out of bed and getting showered is a huge physical effort; getting a pair of socks on, if you have no core strength or stability to balance, is virtually impossible by yourself and if you have no strength in your legs, it is also very difficult to push your feet into your shoes.

We have found that exercise and diet have really helped and even though James was not willing for some time to take responsibility on this level, he now is able to see that it is the only way forward at this present moment. In the meantime, he has now got a family friend Anthony Delamare (who is a personal trainer) on board to help him.

Other symptoms that no one else is generally aware of is incontinence of both bladder and bowels, so unlike an able-bodied person who can rush to the loo, a disabled person is living in constant fear of humiliation, as they cannot rush anywhere and because the muscles have no strength, accidents can happen at any time. If James does not go to the toilet, he often stays trapped indoors the whole day, which for a generally gregarious and very sociable person is very frustrating and leads to anger and resentment, which is perfectly understandable, though hard to live with at times.

We manage without outside carers at the moment and hope to continue to be able to do so for the foreseeable future, as for a grown man to have people outside the family seeing him so helpless is humiliating

and would only make him feel worse.

On the plus side, he is still as ambitious as ever, and has lots of projects on the go, which no doubt will prove successful and keep his mind active and positive.

The Sha

Once Maze Hill was sold, I googled to try and find a healthy holiday. I did not know what exactly I was looking for, but felt desperate to find a place where James could get holistic treatments and was hopeful that we may help reverse his condition. I found The Sha in Alicante, a beautiful macrobiotic spa which had a great reputation for very high quality macrobiotic food as well as shiatsu massage and colon cleansing. Incredibly expensive but I thought worth giving it a try and we booked a ten-day stay.

The people were very friendly and the macrobiotic food was excellent, but in all honesty, I found the place a little clinical and I sensed James was pretty bored. The problem with being disabled is you cannot do most of the things that everyone else can do. For example, I enjoyed the organised walks along the sea front and also Nordic walking as well as yoga and Qi gong. The only thing James could do with ease was swim. He did also enjoy the shiatsu massage, which was excellent, but after the first colon cleanse, nothing could persuade him to have another one. I cannot say I enjoy them, but think that they are extremely beneficial from time to time, especially if you have digestive problems. I was also happy to lose about half a stone and would happily go back for more treatments, if it cost a lot less. It is popular with Madonna, Naomi Campbell and Gwyneth Paltrow, so the prices they charge are in keeping with the clientele they attract. Many people go there to re-charge their batteries and lose weight and if you need help with getting back on track with a healthy eating programme, it is a great place.

Moving from our old house was pretty traumatic for the whole family, especially James, but finding our present home, which is wonderfully historic and has fantastic grounds and a communal club with swimming pool, sauna, steam and gym was indeed a huge blessing. Sadly though, James fell in the club a few times and unfortunately (even though we have bought our flat outright and pay service charges) some people do not think that they should make the club facilities disabled-friendly (at least they are not in any hurry to do so). This is very sad in this day and age, when you would think that most people would consider this essential and normal.

James has been waiting six years for them to put up handrails and they still have not. It is not only sad, but obviously his health has deteriorated more rapidly than it would have, had he been swimming regularly. His top body is still very strong and it would have helped his core stability greatly. Recently, we have found that there is a club at Eltham swimming baths for disabled people; the Lion Club. James is now a member and they come to our home and collect him once a week, which is a great help.

In the meantime, I also have to shoulder more (no pun intended), and literally have to use arnica balm and Biofreeze every day on my neck, shoulders and lower back to help alleviate the stress. Just getting the wheelchair in and out of the car is a heavy load for a woman, and doing all the physical work for two people is a lot to manage by myself; but hopefully a stair lift will be fitted at the entrance to the club, which is just beneath our flat, then James will be swimming again and life will be a lot easier!

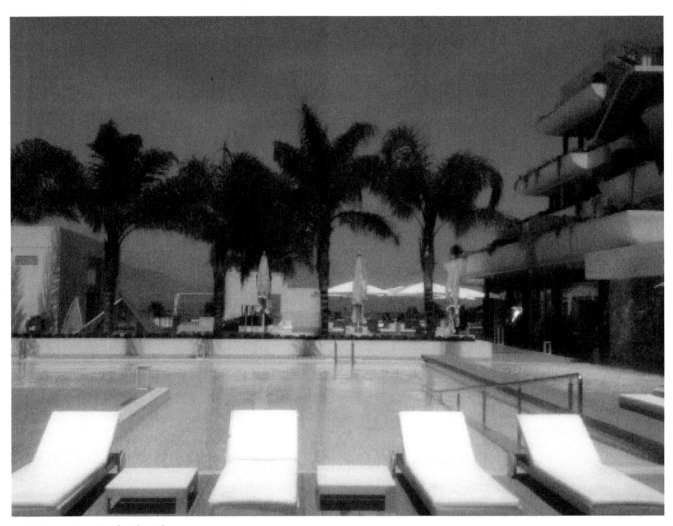

Swimming Pool, The Sha

Balneario de Archena (Holistic Vacation)

We have over the years travelled widely so when James became disabled I had an idea of the sort of location I was looking for for future holidays, and when I found Balneario de Archena, near Murcia in Spain, I was really delighted. We have since been there three times and each year it gets better. I was looking for a place with guaranteed sunshine as well as health treatments and health foods and I do not think we could find better than this.

Spanish people, in general, still eat a very traditional diet, but at Balneario, they went out of their way to try and accommodate our taste in food and would cook brown rice for us every day, grill us vegetables and cook us fresh fish. There was always plenty of fresh fruit, salad and fruit de seco (dried fruit and nuts available). There was some confusion from time to time, so we did have our Fawlty Towers moments, when it felt like we were being served by Manuel; but we had a good chuckle about it. The more they got used to us, the better the service became so it has improved greatly since we started going there and the friendliness of all the staff makes up for the language barrier. They do also have Spanish and English menus but I prefer to keep practising my Spanish. When in Rome…

The flight is short and we get collected from the airport, arranged by the hotel, which takes so much pressure from James, as driving is now very stressful for him. The rooms we have are fantastic and it really feels like home from home. We have a very large bedroom and a dressing room plus large bathroom with easy access for the wheelchair. Jessie, one of the staff, a lovely young woman, organises everything for us, and sort out any queries if we have any and speaks fluent English, which is a great help.

On arrival everyone has a consultation with the doctor, who fortunately does speak a little English. This is so they can decide what treatments are best for you. James mentioned that extra rails in the shower and by the toilet would be helpful as he could not balance and the following day the doctor arranged for them to be put up for him. Fantastic service and made a huge difference to our holiday, alleviating a lot of stress.

As Balneario is set in a conservation area it is wonderful not to have car fumes and to be in a lush location surrounded by river and trees. I would take long morning walks in the early hours, and do a vocal practice in peace, knowing that I was not disturbing anyone, which was wonderful.

Because there are no chemicals in the water, it is fantastic for the skin. We find by the end of our holiday we are positively glowing. We get daily treatments of hot mud and Archena massages and we also tried the flotation therapy, which is really heavenly. The old hotel that we stay in has amazing history and was built at the end of the nineteenth century. With its Moorish architecture it has a lot of old world charm and authentic character.

The outdoor area is wonderful for soaking up the sunshine and has a large outdoor swimming pool and also indoor pool with plenty of sun beds. There is also a restaurant by the poolside as well as a thermal pool which has water jets; a cold plunge pool, lemon water pool, salt therapy which is truly blissful as well as sauna, steam and massages are also available.

There are also outdoor pools with sun loungers and if you are severely disabled they also have lifts to get you in and out of the water.

In the evening after supper, we enjoyed listening to music by the dancing area outdoors while sitting under the massive palm and other ancient trees in this area. Truly relaxing and peaceful. We look forward to returning again this year.

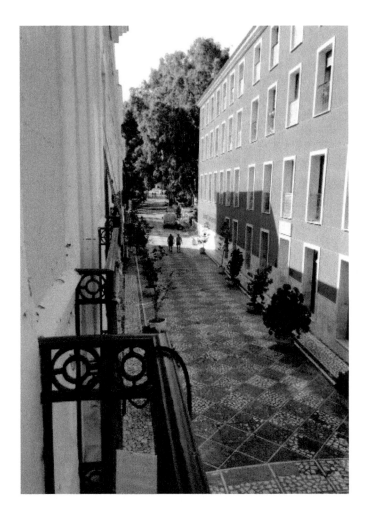

Balneario de Archena

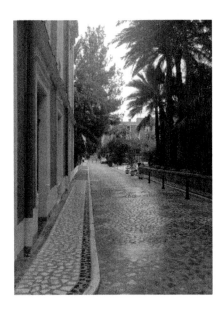

Radisson Blue Malta

We had not been home very long after our holiday at Balneario, when I got a call from Radisson Blu, Malta, part of the Hilton Hotel group. We had builders in while we were away in Spain, making the en suite bathroom disabled-friendly for James. Travelling is always stressful and when you have washing to sort out as well as the builder's mess, you feel like you need another holiday. So when Radisson offered such a good deal and had such excellent disability facilities, I could not resist and we booked and found that it totally lived up to our expectations.

We were met at the airport and our taxi driver Jonathan was really friendly and incredibly helpful. This makes such a huge difference to us as travelling with disability can be very stressful. We got chatting and I asked him where I could get rice or almond milk and even though it was almost 8 pm, he stopped at a small shop en route to the hotel, got them to stay open for me and even though we had no cash on us, came into the shop with me and said I could get whatever I needed and give him the money once we arrived at the hotel where I could get cash. Amazing!

The rest of the holiday continued in much the same way with everyone very hands-on, cheerful and helpful. We enjoyed swimming daily and I was ecstatic to be able to swim in the sea (it had been several years). We went on a coach trip into town and the tourist guide and passengers alike were all willing to help James. He also swam every day in the pool and we both enjoyed fantastic massage treatments;

Aleksandra Zimmerman was particularly caring with her Hawaiian temple massage, called Lomi Lomi Nui. Our apartment was spacious with great facilities and a lovely balcony overlooking the sea. Bliss!

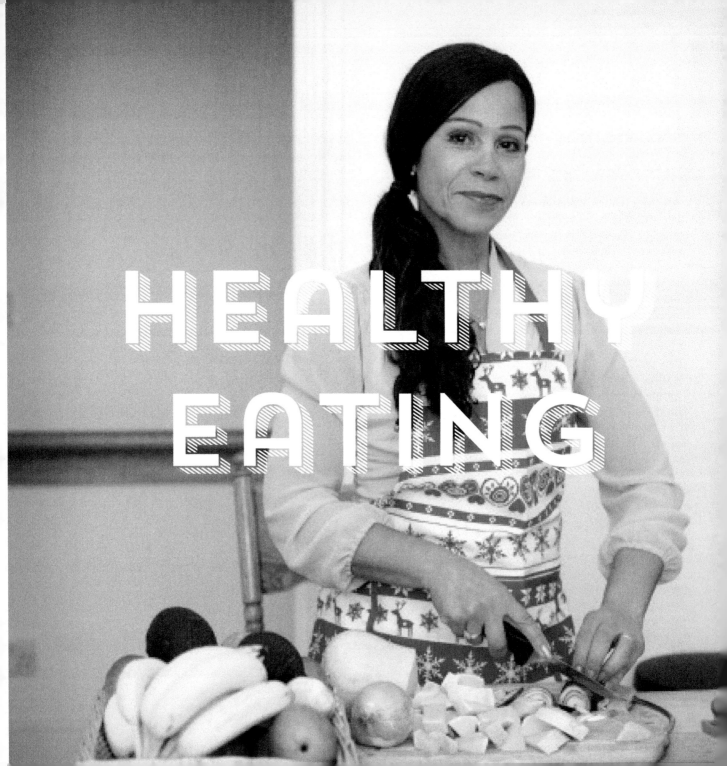

Healthy Eating

Here are some helpful tips for healthy eating, diet and exercise.

Whole Grains

It is good to realise there are many different types of flour but the most nutritious ones are made with whole grain. This means it has the roughage that helps it pass through the digestive system more easily, and it contains more nutrients. White flour is mainly just starch, and unless organic or high quality flour, it often has been bleached!

Gluten free flour is better for us who are gluten intolerant. Ancient flour like spelt flour does contain some gluten, as does rye, but they are both easier to digest. Corn and brown rice flour are both gluten free as is potato flour but if you are like me, and prone to arthritis, it is best you avoid potato flour.

Breakfast – Fruity, Creamy Cereal

2 cups soya milk unsweetened
2 cups almond milk
1 or 2 tablespoons raisins
2 apples
1 pear
10 strawberries
Half a cup of ground almonds
2 tablespoons, unsweetened soya yogurt (optional)

Method

Pour liquid into large airtight container. Wash and chop fruit into small pieces. Add all ingredients to liquid. Keep in fridge until ready to serve. Before serving, cinnamon can be added or rice or cornflakes to make a crunchy texture, or crunchy topping. See recipe.

Lean Cuisine-Salmon and Miso Soup

2 pieces cooked salmon

2 onions

Half a broccoli

2 spring onions, finely diced

1 clove garlic

2 teaspoons grated ginger

1 tablespoon miso

4 cups water

1 teaspoon oil (optional)

Salad leaves/fresh basil (optional)

Method

Crush garlic. Dice onions. Sauté together in frying pan. Wash and break broccoli into small pieces add. Place lid until soft. Transfer all ingredients to pot. Add water. Add pre-cooked salmon and ginger and lastly when salmon is heated, and just before serving, add miso. I enjoy with salad leaves added, but you can just garnish with basil before serving or spring onions if preferred, and drizzle oil on top.

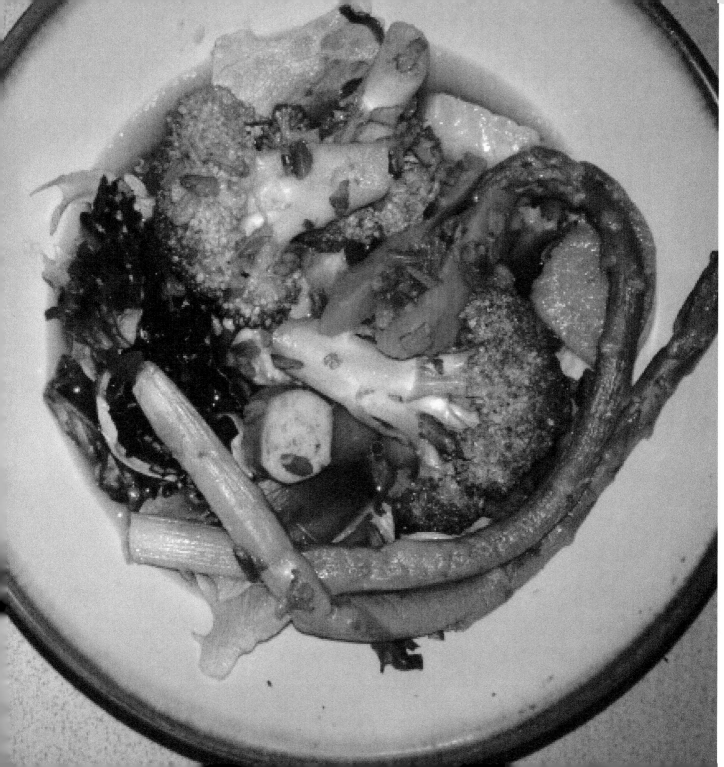

Black Rice with Smoked Tofu, Veg, Salad, with Hummus and Toast

1 cup cooked black rice

1 cup cooked veg

1 packet smoked tofu

Salad /salad dressing

Hummus

Toast

Method

Heat rice, veg and tofu in frying pan with a little oil. Add soy sauce or tamari to flavour. Herbs can be added of desired. Simmer and pace lid on top. While it is heating prepare salad. Put on plates with dressing. Prepare toast. Put hummus on plates then add rice dish. Garnish with fresh basil and serve.

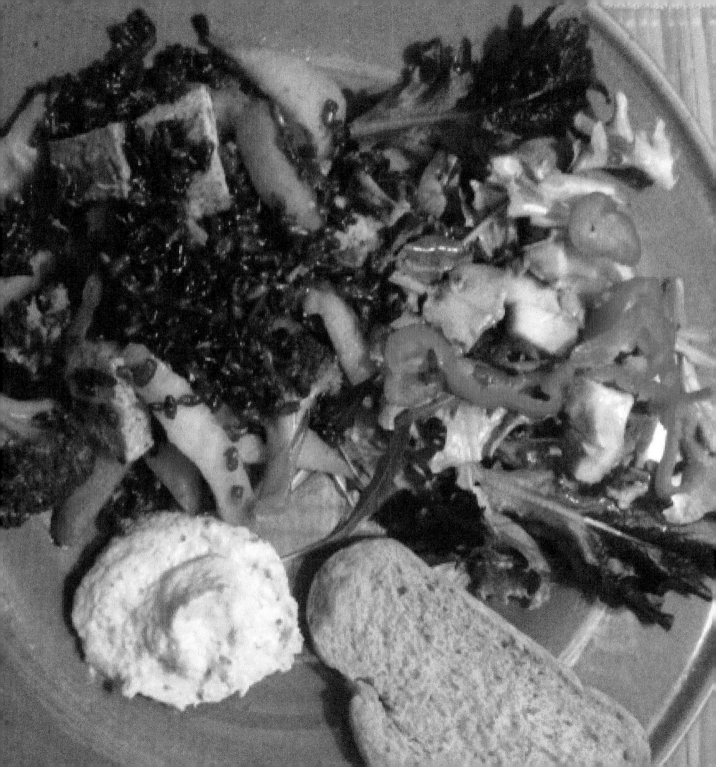

Freshly Baked Salmon and Cod

2 pieces fresh salmon

2 or 3 pieces fresh cod

1 tablespoon oil

1 tablespoon soy sauce or tamari

Garlic

1 teaspoon sweet tarragon

Method

Heat oven to mid temperature/around 200 degrees. Crush garlic in pot. Add oil, soy sauce and herbs. Wash fish and place on baking tray. To make easier to clean, cover tray with silver foil, place fish on tray and coat evenly with dressing. When oven us hot place fish on middle shelf and cook for approx. 15 mins. Serve with rice, salad and veg can be garnished with roast almonds or cashews before serving.

(You can also use sea bass if preferred!)

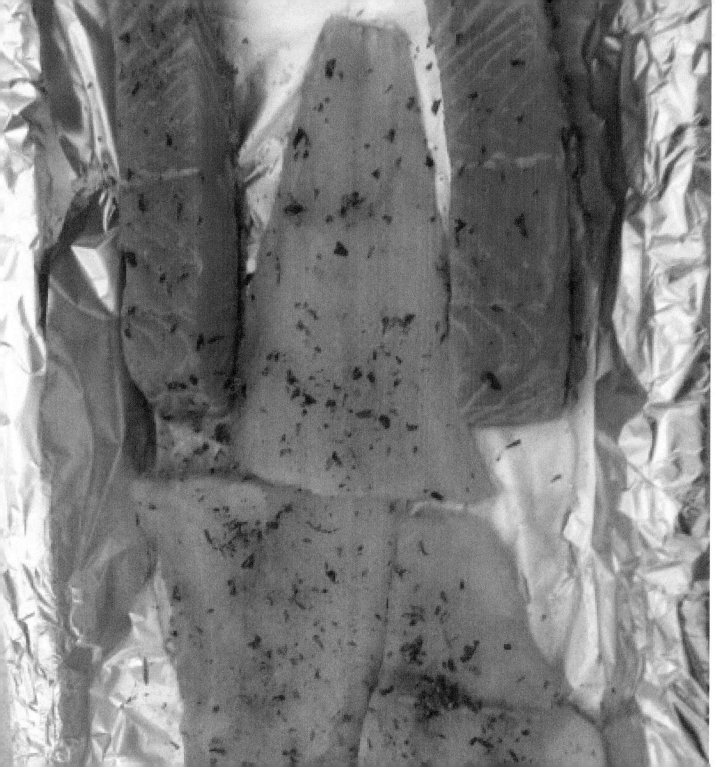

Garlic Asparagus

2 packets asparagus

1 clove garlic

1 tablespoon sunflower oil

1 dessertspoon tamari or soy sauce

1 tablespoon sesame seeds

Method

Wash the asparagus. Cut of about an inch from the end of each piece. Crush garlic. Heat in frying pan, add asparagus and a little water. Simmer with lid on. When almost cooked but still al dente, coat with soy sauce. Sesame seeds can be sprinkled on top before serving.

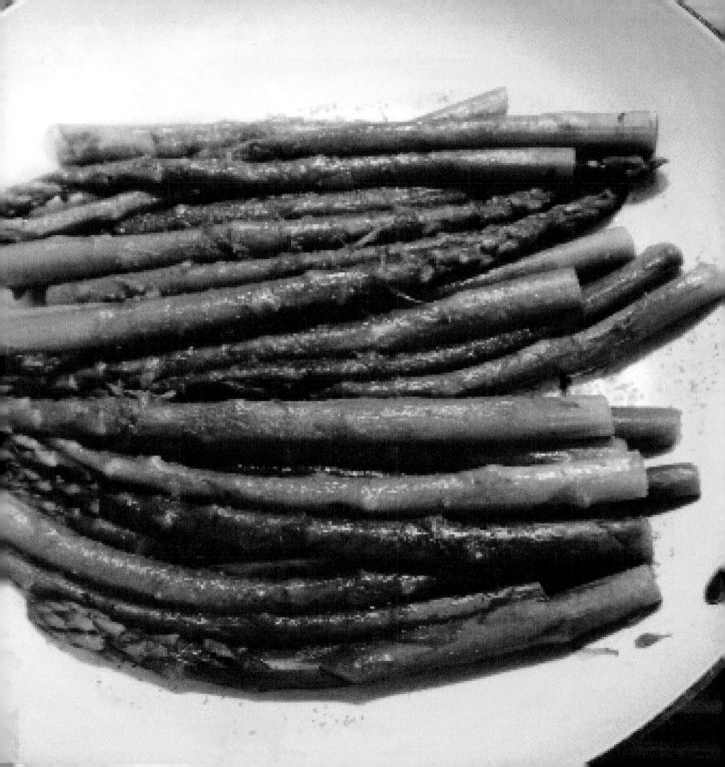

Sticky Black Rice

Sticky black rice makes a wonderful change from brown rice. It is high in antioxidants, easy to digest and delicious. The Chinese emperors used to eat this rice because of its nutritional value.

Method

Cook the same as brown rice. One cup of rice to two cups of water.

Wash rice, put in pot, add water, and bring to boil, simmer until all water is absorbed. Sea salt may be added during cooking if desired.

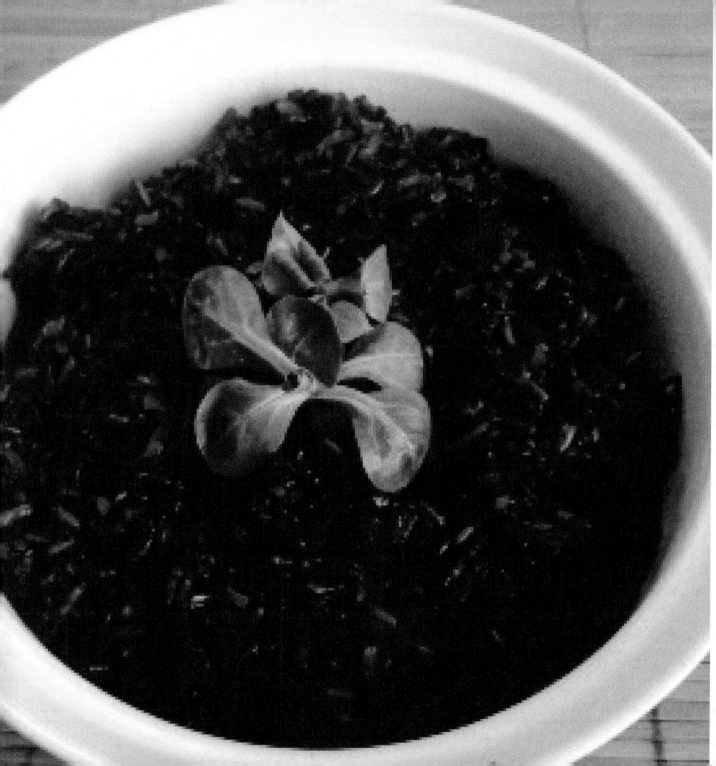

Sautéed Vegetables

2 leeks

2 carrots

1 broccoli head

2 parsnips

1 clove garlic

1 tablespoon sunflower oil

1 tablespoon soy sauce or tamari

Method

Wash and cut vegetables. Crush garlic and heat in frying pan. Add vegetables putting broccoli at top as they cook quicker. Add a little water. Bring to boil. Place lid on pan and simmer. When still slightly al dente, remove from heat and add soy sauce. Herbs can be added if desired. Also before serving, a handful of tamari roasted cashews can be added or roasted sunflower and pumpkin seeds!

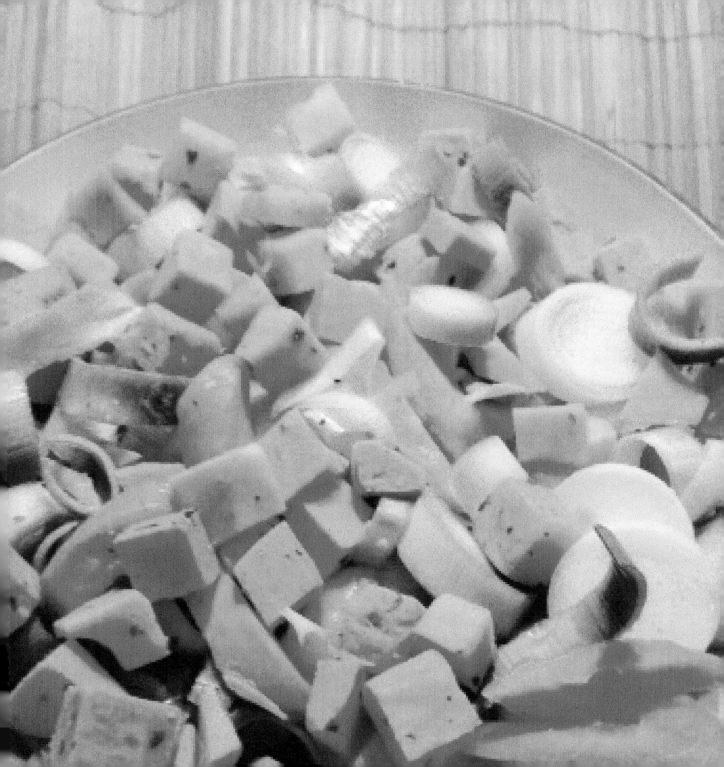

Sautéed Veg with Tofu

2 leeks

2 carrots

1 broccoli head

2 parsnips

1 clove garlic

1 tablespoon sunflower oil

1 tablespoon soy sauce or tamari

1 block of tofu

Method

Follow method for the previous recipe only take block of tofu and steam, add tablespoon soy sauce or tamari and add to vegetables once they are cooked. Also delicious served with roast south almonds (available from SeeWoo, the Chinese supermarket); they have no skin on them, so perfect for roasting.

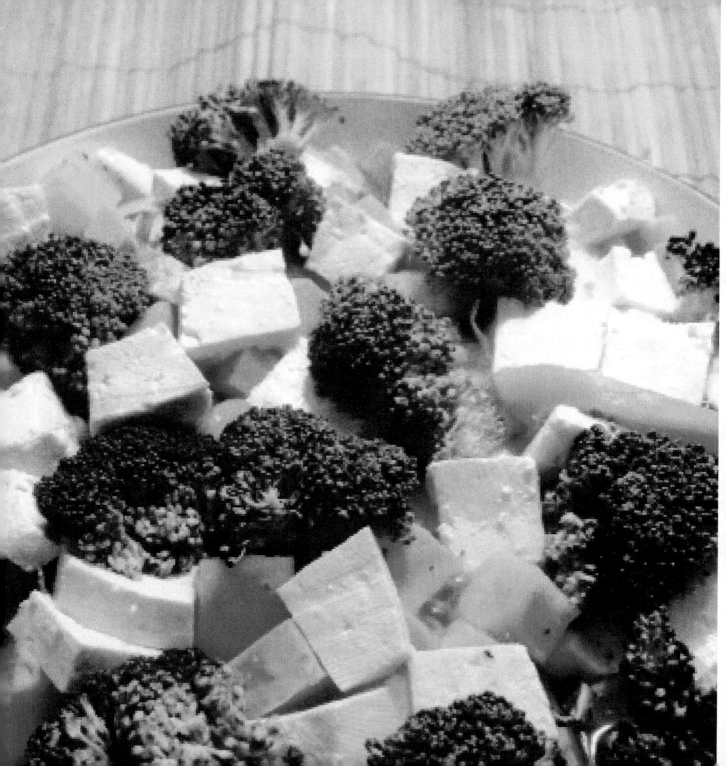

Long Stemmed Broccoli with Fine Green Beans and Roast South Almonds

1 packet fine green beans

1 packet long stemmed broccoli

1 clove of garlic

1 desert spoon soy sauce

1 desert spoon sunflower oil

1 handful roast south almonds

Quarter of a red pepper sliced finely for garnish

Method

Crush garlic and heat oil in frying pan. Add garlic when hot then broccoli and beans. Add a little water and bring to boil, then place lid and simmer. When cooked to al dente, add soy sauce or tamari and before serving garnish with almonds and peppers.

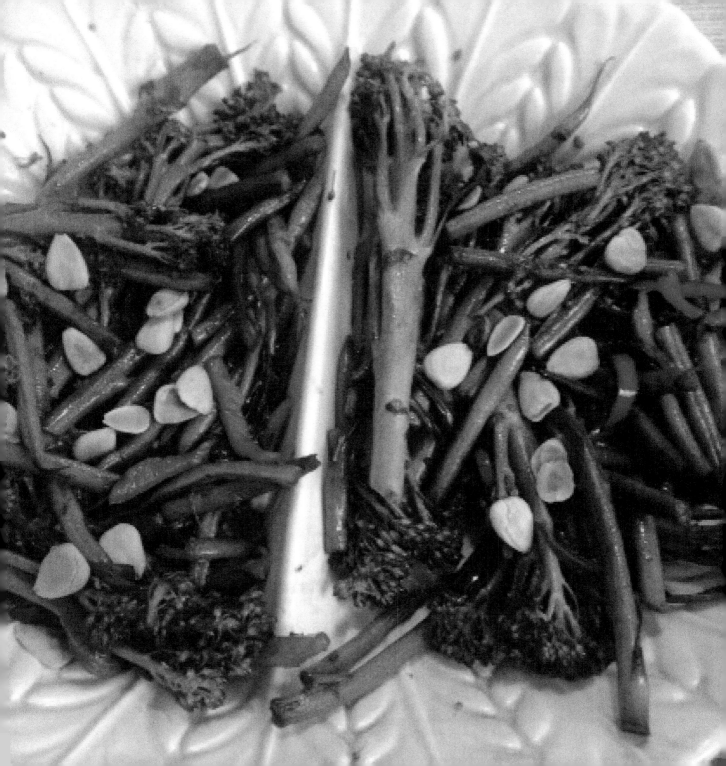

Sushi

Nori seaweed 1 packet (you will probably only use 2 or 3 sheets)

Softly cooked brown rice, which is slightly sticky, 1 pot, though you will not use it all

Filling of your choice:

Avocado

Cucumber

Smoked Salmon

You can also buy an organic pickled ginger sushi condiment, perfect for sushi. You just dice a little and add before rolling.

Miso – best to use fairly runny paste by mixing a spoonful in a small pot and adding a small amount of water

Method

Lay a sheet of nori on the sushi mat. Place around 4 dessertspoons of rice on mat. Leave an inch from the side nearest to you, without rice. Make an indentation along the centre with a chopstick, as this is where the filling will go. Fill firstly with miso paste then you can add sliced avocado or cucumber, or slivers of smoked salmon. When filling has been placed all across the centre, take edge of nori mat and roll tightly. It does take practice and you should dampen the far end with a little water so that it will stick. Once it is rolled into a long sausage roll shape, place on a wooden chopping board and slice into inch size pieces with a very sharp knife. You can arrange on a plate before serving and it's delicious served with a dip.

You can make a dip simply with soy sauce, water, grated ginger or daikon radish. Make according to your taste!

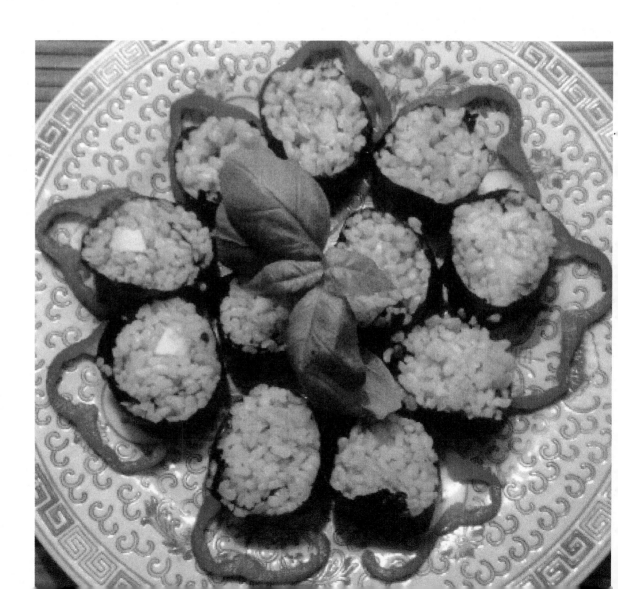

Roasted Sunflower and Pumpkin Seeds

1 cup raw sunflower seeds

1 cup raw pumpkin seeds

1 tablespoon tamari or soy sauce

Method

Heat oven to 200 degrees. Place seeds evenly on baking tray. When oven is hot, place on middle shelf and bake until golden brown. Check after 10 minutes. If not cooked, then rotate with spoon so they all cook evenly. When ready, remove from oven and coat lightly with tamari or soy sauce.

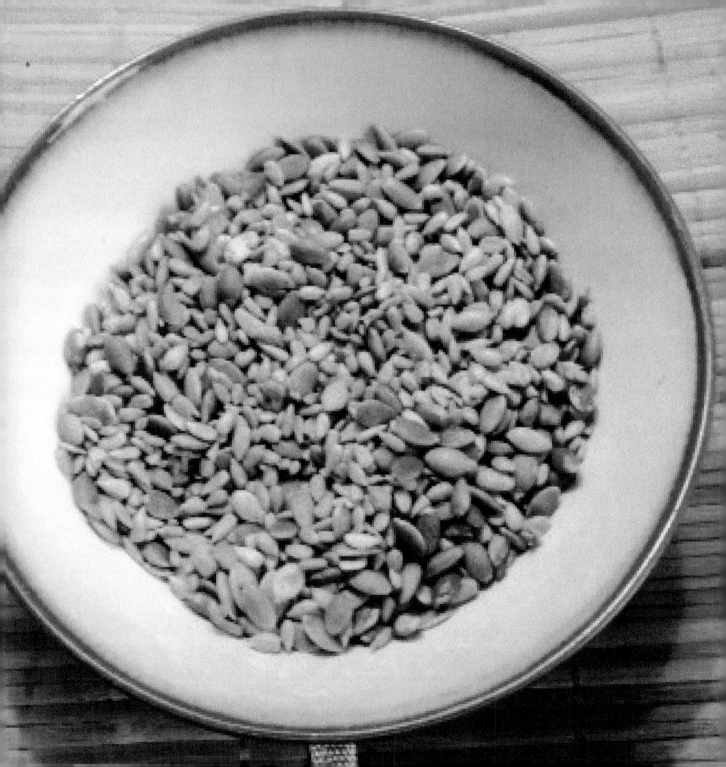

Summertime Snack for Two

Two pears

6 strawberries

1 handful walnuts

1 handful raisins

2 handfuls crunch topping

2 tablespoons cinnamon if desired

Method

Wash fruit. Cut and place on 2 dishes. Put a handful of crunchy topping in centre of each dish. Sprinkle walnuts and radians on top. Sprinkle cinnamon on top and serve.

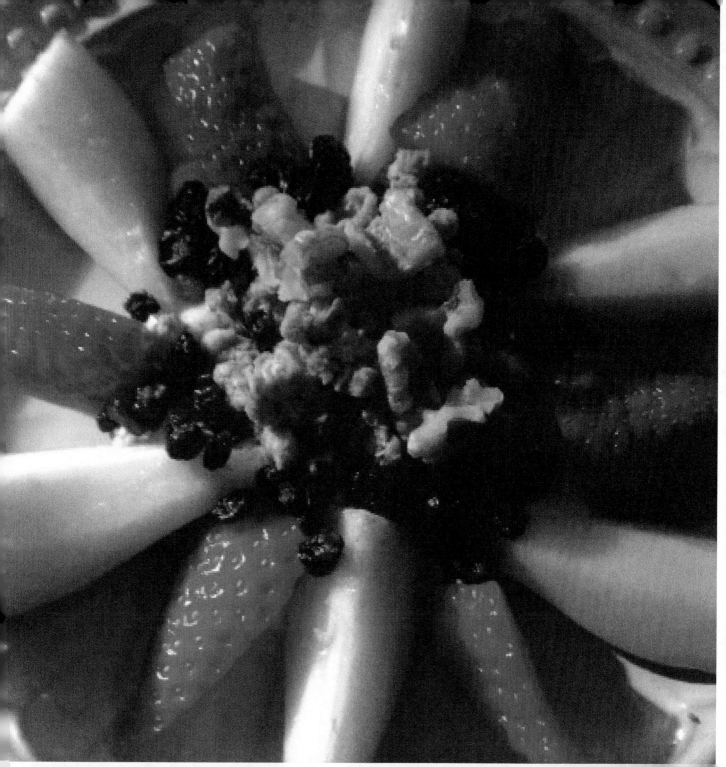

Crunchy Wholewheat and Oat Biscuits

2 cups oats (can be gluten free if preferred)

2 cups whole-wheat self-raising flour (or gluten free flour if preferred)

Quarter cup sunflower oil

A quarter cup of sesame seeds

A quarter cup of raisins

2 teaspoons cinnamon (optional)

2 tablespoons agave syrup

Water to mix

A handful of walnuts (optional)

Method

Heat oven to 200 degrees. Mix all ingredients in bowl thoroughly, adding water a little at a time until mixture binds together easily. Press flat in large baking tray and then divide with knife into biscuit size pieces. When oven is hot place on middle shelf and bake for approx. 20 mins until golden.

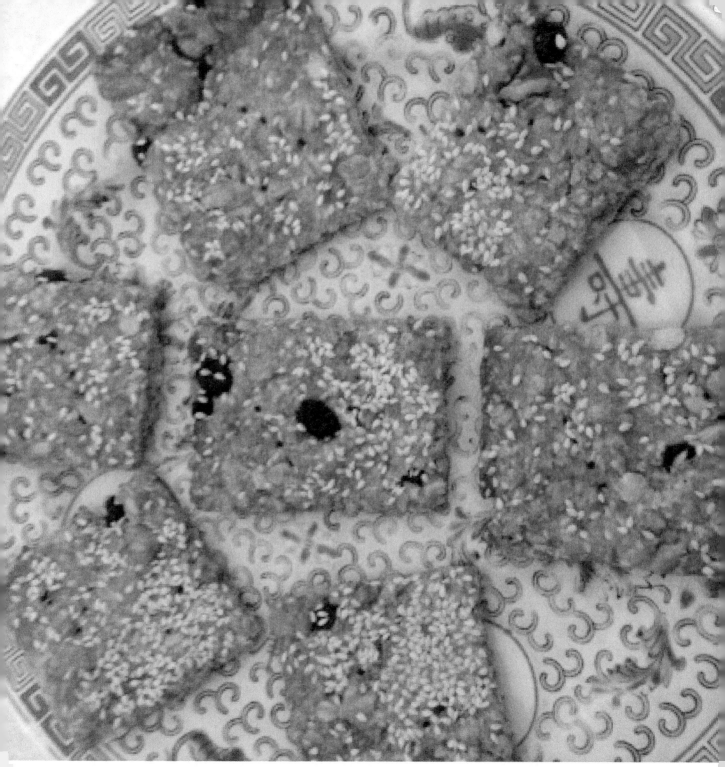

Jam Turnovers

Using the same pastry as for mince pies

Method

Filling

St Dalfour raspberry jam

4 pears

Wash and cut pears. Heat in pan, cook until soft. Add four tablespoons of jam when cool.

Roll out party and cut into 5-inch squares. Place filling in centre, then wet edges with water and fold into a triangular shape.

Heat oven to 200 degrees and when oven is hot, bake until golden brown. Delicious served with ice cream, yoghurt or custard as suggested above.

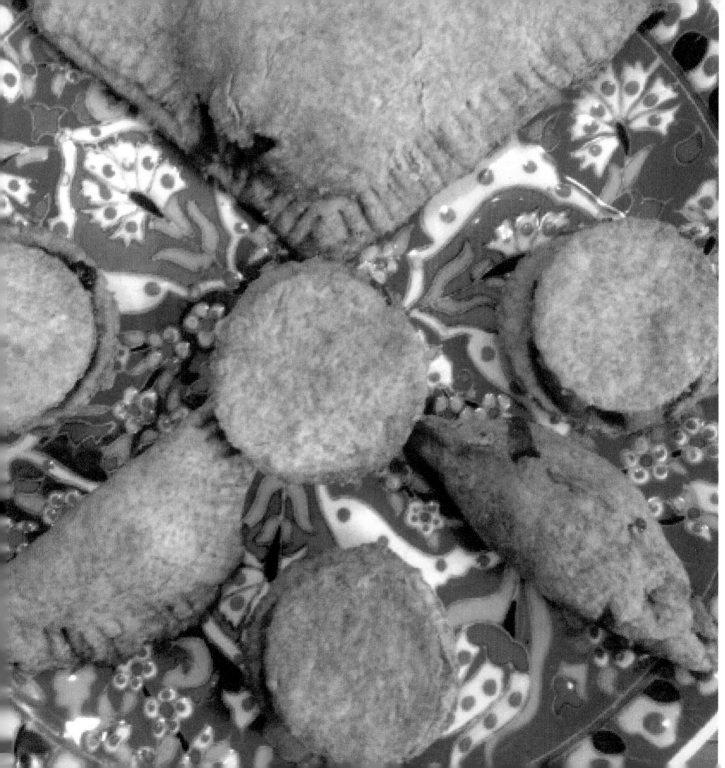

Raspberry and Apple Flan

Using the same pastry as for the turnovers.

Filling

St Dalfour raspberry jam

4 apples

Method

Exactly the same as for the turnovers, just roll the pastry into a large flan dish and bake until golden. Fill with cooked filling and serve with custard cream or yogurt as suggested previously. Soya or coconut being preferable to the dairy variety. You can also use St Dalfour blackberry jam instead of raspberry. Enjoy experimenting!

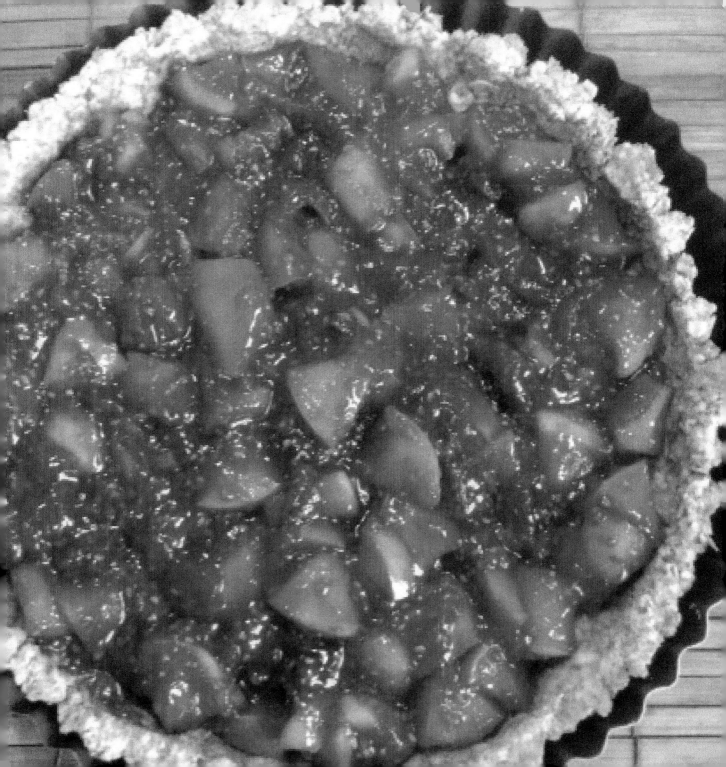

Mince Pies

Pastry

2 cups whole-wheat or spelt flour

1 teaspoon of doves baking powder

Quarter cup of sunflower oil

Pinch of sea salt

1 tablespoon fruit sugar or agave syrup

Water to mix

Filling

1 jar organic mincemeat from health food shop (I prefer the unsweetened, which is very sweet)

2 apples

Method

Heat oven to 200 degrees

Roll pastry onto floured surface. Use pastry cutter and cut so they will fit neatly into bun tin, grease tin with a little oil. When oven is hot, bake until golden. Then remove and allow cooling on cooling rack.

Wash and core apples. Then place in large pan with a little water and cook until soft. Add the whole jar of mincemeat. Fill each of the pastry bases then roll out rest of pastry and using smaller cutter, cut out pastry to make lids for each pastry base. Bake as before. When cool, place on top of each base! Delicious served with Booja-Booja ice cream or Swedish glaze. This does contain some sugar, though no dairy so I prefer to just use a small quantity. You can also get delicious coconut or chocolate flavoured ice cream from health food shops with no dairy and only a little sweetener. Provamel make delicious sugar free custard, available from Holland and Barrett, or enjoy with plain soya yogurt. I sometimes mix them together, which is equally delicious, and sprinkle with cinnamon. Any leftover pastry can be made into biscuits. Just add raisins and some cinnamon, roll out and bake!

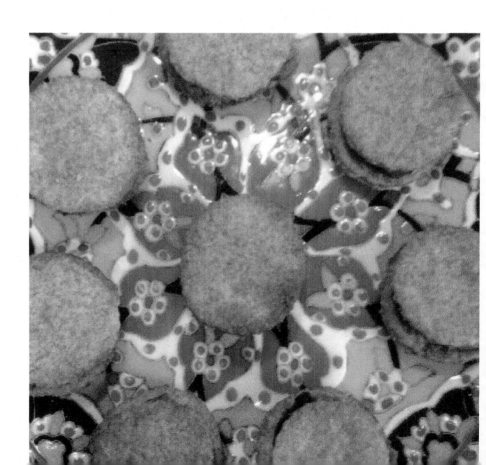

Chocolate Party Biscuits

3 cups of puffed brown rice cereal

Half a bar of Green & Black's chocolate
(milk if for children)

1 tablespoon agave syrup

1 tablespoon almond butter

Method

Melt chocolate in pan, remove from heat and add all the other ingredients and mix thoroughly. Press into greased baking tray then refrigerate. Cut into pieces when cool and serve!

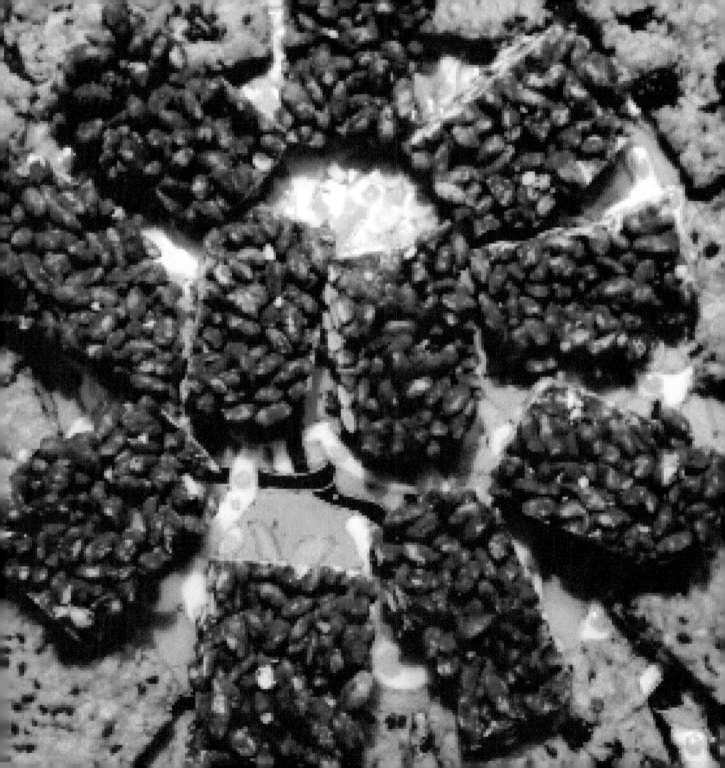

Cheatin' Chocolate Cake

1 packet Hale & Hearty gluten free cake mix

1 cup spelt flour

200g pure margarine (or 6 tablespoons of organic sunflower oil)

2 tablespoons cocoa powder

1 cup almond milk

4 eggs (or Doves baking powder)

2 teaspoons (Doves baking powder)

Filling

St Dalfour jam – black cherry or raspberry work well

Topping

Green & Black's chocolate (I prefer plain but children prefer milk)

Nuts to decorate if desired

Method

Heat oven to 175C. Mix all ingredients together in a bowl really thoroughly until a smooth, creamy consistency (if too stiff, then add a little more almond milk). Grease two baking tins or line them with greaseproof paper (easier to clean and get out of tins).

Pour mixture into tins and bake for 25 mins. Tip onto baking tray and allow cooling. When cool, you can melt chocolate in pot and decorate top. Keep refrigerated until ready to use. Delicious!

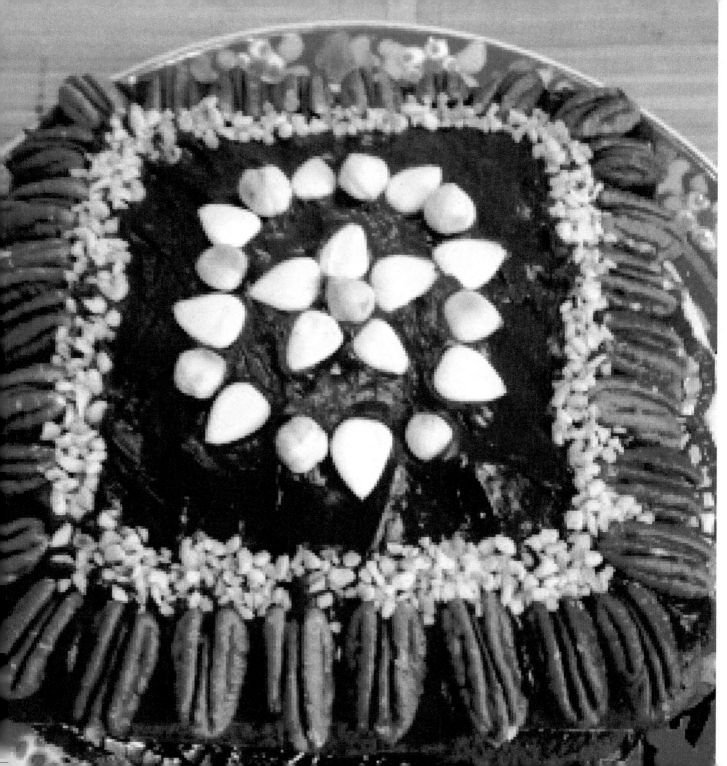

Healthy Snacks

People say do not snack between meals but I always take healthy snacks to eat and I feel it sustains me in a good way. My hours of work can be very long and if one snacks on seeds, nuts, raw veg, i.e. carrot sticks, celery, apples and grapes, it is better than getting ridiculously hungry and then over-eating. Find what suits you best and enjoy. On the recipe pages is a recipe for roast sunflower and pumpkin seeds. I usually mix them with a handful of raisins. You can also mix in walnuts and Brazil nuts, and they are delicious with roast hazelnuts added.

Mums, Pregnancy and Beautiful Baby

This is indeed an incredibly important time in a woman's life; the fact we are graced with the power to bring a life into this world is wonderful, though it can often be a real struggle to balance if one has to work long hours to make ends meet. Hopefully with the help of a loving partner or family, yours will be an enjoyable journey.

Childbirth is not always a pain-free and blissful experience, but the joy usually comes with holding your baby for the first time and realising what a miracle it is.

It is so sad that some women cannot breast feed, but if you can, it is definitely advisable you do so. The body is producing all that milk for a reason, as nature intended for your child to drink, which also helps strengthen and boost the baby's immunity, helps with natural bonding between mum and baby, and also helps you get back into shape a lot faster.

Once the baby is ready to eat solid food, it is really easy to purée your own. It is also way healthier and cost effective and you will know exactly what your child is consuming.

We are led to believe that children should consume lots of sweets, but they are generally better off without them. Many contain colouring and E numbers which can lead to hyperactivity and mood swings, in turn making it harder for them to concentrate on anything for very long, so can be a real problem once they are at school.

Once they get labelled as a slow learner, or not able to concentrate, this can be extremely detrimental to their self-belief. It is much kinder to stick to a healthier diet for their benefit and well-being.

Understandably this can be difficult but will power and determination is important and it does pay off in the end! If they do have a sweet tooth then cook or purée a variety of sweet fruits when they are a toddler and make your own biscuits and cakes when they get older. You can now get a lot more healthy food in the supermarkets, but do check the quantity of sugar used. It is often the first ingredient. You can also buy sweets that are more naturally sweetened, from health food stores. They are a lot more expensive, but as they should just be eaten as treats, hopefully your child will not be consuming masses of them; so overall the cost will not be high.

It will be your decision whether your child takes a packed lunch and I guess that will depend largely on the choices available at the school they will attend. I always preferred Jay, my son, to have a packed lunch. My memory of school dinners was not great and I think in many schools they have deteriorated over the years!

If they have a chance to be involved in creative pursuits from a young age, this is great for them. Dancing, playing musical instruments, and fresh air daily are all wonderful for the spirit. Please remember that education does begin in the home and if you provide them with tools, books, pens, paper, paints, they will use them, be brighter for it and more confident. Way better than dumping them in front of the TV. Also eating as part of a family where possible is a great way of bonding daily. TV dinners can be alienating, whereas if you are sitting around a table together, you are much more likely to communicate with each other, which makes for a happier home life.

Ingredients

Here is a list of wonderful ingredients you will find useful if you wish to eat a wide variety of natural produce.

GRAINS
Brown rice
Brown basmati rice
Black rice
Red rice
Wholewheat couscous

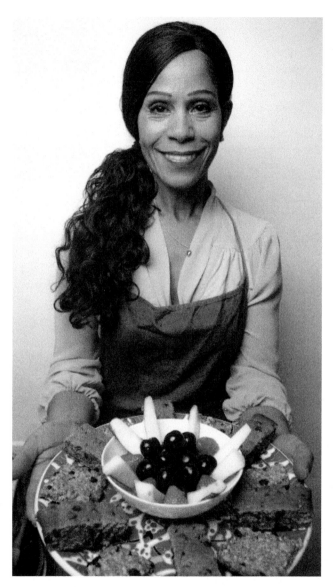

Quinoa
Barley
Corn
Millet
Polenta
Udon noodles
Buckwheat pasta
Brown rice pasta
Vermicelli brown rice pasta (great added to winter soups)
Bean pasta
Amaranth
Corn cakes
Rice cakes
Buckwheat cakes

CEREALS
Puffed brown rice
Organic corn flakes (unsweetened)
Puffed buckwheat

PROTEINS
Spirulina
Tofu
Adzuki beans
Hummus
Tofu sausages
Falafel
Quinoa (the grain with the most protein)

CONDIMENTS
Soy sauce
Tamari
Miso
Harissa paste
Pesto (you can get dairy free if preferred
Manuka honey
St Dalfour jam (just sweetened with apple juice)
Cashew nut butter
Almond butter
Organic sunflower oil (Suma oil can be bought on Amazon in 5-litre bottles, very economical)
Rapeseed oil
Sesame oil
Coconut oil
Kudzu (Japanese organic arrowroot)
Organic cider vinegar (Biona vinegar can also be bought on Amazon in 5-litre bottles, great for detoxing and can be drunk diluted with water to help those with arthritis!)

DRIED FRUITS, NUTS AND SEEDS
Bounce balls, available from health food stores, are packed full of nutrients and great when you are low in and need a quick supply, e.g. before performance sports or dance class.
Raisins
Figs
Dates
Hunza apricots
Dark apricots
Walnuts

Brazil nuts
Hazel nuts
Almonds
South almonds
Pecan nuts
Sunflower seeds
Pumpkin seeds
Back sesame seeds
White sesame seeds
Cinnamon (great for naturally sweetening and for people with diabetes)
Raw cacao nibs (great for satisfying chocolate cravings and energy giving)
Agave syrup
Fruit sugar

SEAWEEDS
Arami
Nori
Kombu (very warming, so great for bodily warmth along with miso in winter months, especially if recovering from illness).

It is also good to stock up on a wide variety of herbs as they add make experimenting interesting when you learn about the different flavours and how to use them. Fresh garlic and ginger are wonderful and great for health especially in the winter months.

BEVERAGES
Lots of water (of course, spring, filtered or bottled is best)

Having a wide variety of herbal teas in your cupboards is useful
Green tea
White tea
Peppermint tea
Rooibos tea
There are many more choices of herb teas available on the market

Soya milk (unsweetened)
Rude brown rice milk
Rude almond milk

If you buy juice it is best to buy non-concentrated and freshly pressed juice. Juicing your own is even better but time does not always allow this. Freshly juiced carrots with fresh ginger are a wonderful way to start the day! Fresh carrots each day help keep sickness at bay. Having consumed a fair amount of wine in my late 20s when was working with musicians in Spain, I have a preference to generally steer clear of alcohol, though I do enjoy the odd glass of champagne over the Christmas period and also for birthday celebrations. Alcohol consumption is an individual decision but best not done habitually for its long-term negative side effects.

Fruits and vegetables that are better to consume are ones that are seasonal, especially in winter months as these are ones that give our body more warmth. Carrots, parsnips, onions, swedes, turnips, leeks, and beetroot all help to keep the body warm through the cold winter months and help boost immunity. I love to use a lot of garlic and fresh ginger in the winter months as well; this helps ward off colds and infection.

I mentioned Hunza apricots earlier and just want to add that the Hunza people, who live in the Himalayas, generally live to over 100 years old. Their diet is mainly vegetarian. The Hunza apricot, which is a large part of their diet, is not as sweet as the dried apricots that we usually consume and is denser and said to have a lot of healing properties. If you are interested, you can google more about the Hunza people.

Likewise the Blue Zone people (a term used to identify a demographic or geographic area of the world where people live longer than average lives) are said to have astonishing longevity; again, they generally consume little meat and mainly fresh produce. There has to be something in it. The food we consume is after all what nourishes our bodies, minds and the quality of our blood. Google for more information!

Useful Supplements

Here is a list of natural supplements that you may find useful to incorporate into your diet. When we are younger and in perfect health, we should be able to get all our nutrients from the food we eat. As we get older, however, many of us find that energy levels are depleted. I do supplement my diet and find it extremely helpful, especially as my hours of work can be extremely long and also because I am carrying the physical load for two people. Everybody has different needs, so you have to decide what is best for you. I would absolutely recommend calcium for women going through menopause especially if, like myself, you

prefer a mainly vegan diet. Without it, the bones can become extremely brittle.

Using good quality oil for cooking and drizzling on salads can make a huge difference to your general health and well-being; preferably organic and unrefined. It is also worth looking into homeopathic remedies and also essential oils, for their healing power is immense. You can google information online or see an experienced practitioner for advice.

A good quality multi-vitamin
Spirulina (powdered sea algae) – this can be made into smoothies by adding LINWOOD mix and brown rice milk or almond milk. A great way to start the day.
Gingko biloba – good for memory and circulation
Calcium – good for bones, teeth, hair and nails
Vitamin D – good for skin, hair and nails
Vitamin B – important building blocks for the body, especially during illness or pregnancy
Glucosamine supplement – good for arthritis – one that includes cider vinegar is especially helpful
Ginseng – good for energy
Echinacea – good for boosting the immune system
MSM powder – great for colon cleansing
Fish oil supplement or krill oil
Vitamin E – great for healing skin or any cuts
Arnica cream – great for healing bruising
Green tea – an antioxidant and great energy boost
Argan oil – great for hair
Biotin – for hair and nails
COQ 10 – good for healing heart as well as gum disease
Olbas oil – great for clearing nasal congestion and

you can add a drop or two to boiling hot water and cover your head with a towel to relieve a blocked nose.

I have also found a fantastic facial serum called 180 hyaluronic acid which I have found works wonders for my skin. It's best to buy the extra strength one and use with a high quality natural face cream.

A great home remedy for whitening teeth is putting a teaspoon of Dove organic baking powder in a small pot and adding a few drops of organic apple cider vinegar. It will froth up; as it does so, dip your toothbrush into the mix and brush vigorously. You will find your teeth much brighter and gleaming afterwards.

Other useful products to have in your medicine cupboard

Tea tree oil – natural antiseptic
Tea tree oil cream – natural antiseptic cream
Kalms – tablets that contain valerian, which helps one sleep when restless (no-additive herb)
Rescue remedy – great for alleviating stress
Rescue night remedy – great for restless nights
Bio gel
Aloe vera gel
Organic toothpaste (Dr Organic)
Organic shea butter can be bought at Amazon, in large tubs. Useful for making own creams and great for softening skin.

You can make your own mouth wash by diluting tea tree oil, a couple of teaspoons, adding a tablespoon or two of sunflower oil, a couple of teaspoons of clove oil and a teaspoon of sea salt. Fill the rest of bottle with water and shake vigorously before using. Hold in your mouth for a good five to ten minutes or more, and then rinse your mouth thoroughly.

Finding a good shiatsu practitioner and also acupuncturist is extremely advantageous to wellbeing, especially if you are suffering from illness and don't wish to take chemical medicine. You can google to find out where your local practitioners are.

You can also make your own natural creams at a fraction of the price of shop-bought ones. I buy organic shea butter in a very large quantity online then experiment mixing MSM powder, organic aloe vera, then adding a few drops of an essential oil. Adding lemon balm makes a lovely scent and it is also very healing and nourishing for the skin. I gave a small pot to a man at work who had problematic joints in his hands and he was delighted that it healed them; since using it, he has not had any more problems. This gives me a wonderful feeling! There are lots of different essential oils and they all have different healing powers. Google for information and enjoy experimenting. You can buy little stainless steel pots with airtight lids online on the Amazon website. Perfect for storing the cream in. Enjoy!

CHAPTER 10

Flexible Body, Flexible Mind

I believe the two things really do go hand in hand, and even if you have not been exercising as much as you would like to or feel you should, there is no time like the present moment.

I have also recently discovered Danceworks, near Bond Street tube station, which is a wonderful dance school that also has singing classes. All the classes are at a very reasonable rate. The beauty is that you can just drop in, as and when you please; you do not have to book in advance. All the classes that I have tried so far are excellent, and the teachers great fun and exceptionally experienced as well as hard working. It is fantastic value for money and a great atmosphere throughout the building!

I also attend an open mike, which is really good fun, every Tuesday night upstairs at The Haggerston pub in Hackney. Singing is wonderful for the spirit and it's great to hear all the different styles of creativity from all the performers. Phil Ramercon, who is a very experienced and proficient musician and teacher, runs it. If you wish to take part in performing, get there early and Phil will put your name down on the list. Enjoy!

As food nourishes mind, body and soul, choosing wisely means our bodies will work more efficiently, be more supple and strong and we will have more energy. Of course our heritage and natural constitution at birth will play a large part in our physical ability, but the quality of all we consume will also play a large part in how physically fit we are. The more nutritious our diet, the better equipped we will be to live life fully.

Exercising daily is also really important as it increases blood flow and brainpower as well as stamina. Choosing exercises that suit our natural ability and age is equally as important as doing exercises that we enjoy.

I love swimming, which I do usually twice a week, and practise yoga daily, usually around 15 minutes. I also take a singing class once a week and dance classes twice a week and enjoy walking. This may sound like a lot but because of my early dance training (in my teens), which also included ballet training, it suits my constitution and makes me feel happy. Muscles also have memory, so mine are well equipped for this much exercise and keep me strong enough to manage my husband's disability and lift his wheelchair in and out of the car without causing strain or injury.

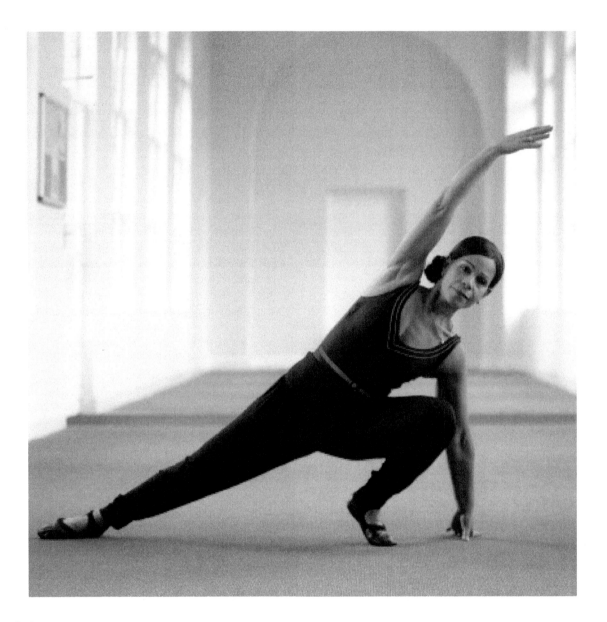

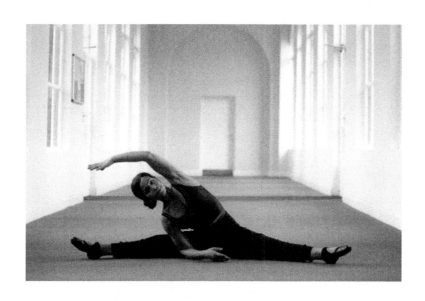

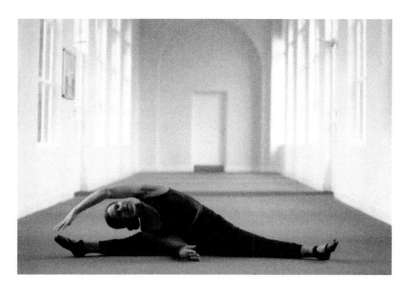

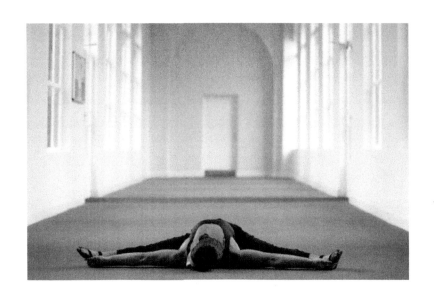

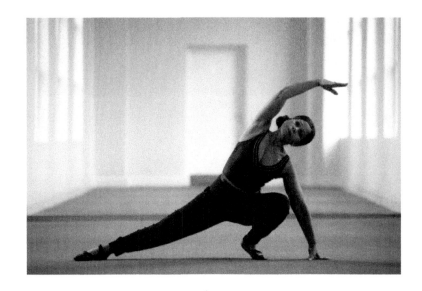

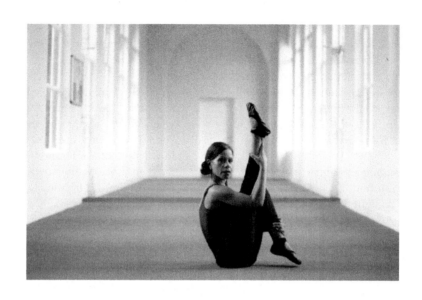

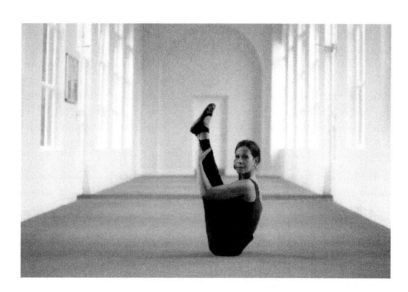

Here are five simple exercises that can be done at home daily. It is better to exercise for 20 minutes each day than two hours one day a week, as you build up more stamina with little and often. If you find them too easy, then just increase the amount or add your own to these. The important thing to remember is to keep good posture, breathe freely, and if you feel fatigue, rest in between. Rome was not built in a day.

1) Squats: standing upright in the kitchen. Hold on to side unit with both hands, facing it, with legs together and back straight. Bend knees and lower yourself down as far as possible, into a low squat. If you cannot go down very low, no worries, you will get there with practice. Count to five then straighten up. Repeat x 5.

2) Leg swings: facing forwards so you are holding on with one hand, swing outside leg as high as you can without bending it. Lower it down and swing it backwards. Repeat x 5 then turn and lift your other leg. Repeat x 5.

3) Cat stretch: lie on your stomach; push up with bent knees so your body is in a table posture. Then arch your back and count to five then hollow your back and count to five. Repeat x 5.

4) Cycling exercise: if you have a carpeted area or yoga mat, lie down on your back and make a cycling action with your legs for a long as you can manage. When you have finished, rest with your knees pulled in to your chest.

5) Skiing exercise: from standing, raise your arms straight and over your head, then swing them forward at the same time bending your knees, imagine you are going down a ski slope. Swing your arms back up and repeat x 5.

With all these exercises, it is important to remember to breathe! Playing music can also really help motivate you, and the rhythm of the music can help inspire you as well. Make sure you relax and rest if you need to when you have finished. If my muscles are feeling fatigued, I like nothing better than a hot bath to help relax my limbs. This usually puts them right but I also use bio gel for more severe aches and pains.

I hope you have enjoyed reading my story and find my health tips useful. If you want to take it one step further and have a larger understanding as to how large consumptions of meat have an extremely negative effect on the world as a whole, please google Cowspiracy. My stepdaughter, Aliyah, suggested my husband read Cowspiracy. He has done, and it has already opened his mind and changed his outlook, which is wonderful. By reading this information you will internalise and understand the impact that our individual actions have, and discover how you can change the reality of the whole world and have more empathy and compassion with those in third world countries where there are food shortages.

An open mind is an open heart. We really do have the power within each of us to change the whole world, if we try to and make a responsible choice to do so.

The power is ours!

Simone

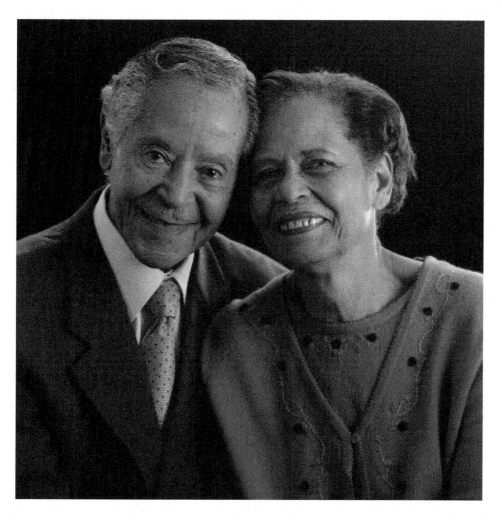

And special thanks to my parents too.

Lightning Source UK Ltd.
Milton Keynes UK
UKOW07f0011211016

285749UK00002B/16/P

9 781911 110835